CH

D0250982

The Naughty Diet

The Naughty Diet

The 10-Step Plan to
Eat and Cheat Your Way
to the Body You Want

Melissa Milne

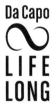

Da Capo

LIFE
LONG

A Member of the Perseus Books Group

Editorial production by *Marrathon Production Services*. www.marrathon.net

Designed by Joe Heroun

Library of Congress Cataloging-in-Publication Data
Name: Milne, Melissa, author.
Title: The naughty diet : the 10-step plan to eat and cheat your way to the
body you want / by Melissa Milne.
Description: Boston, MA : Da Capo Lifelong Books, a member of the Perseus
Books Group, [2016] | Includes bibliographical references and index.
Identifiers: LCCN 2016003903 (print) | LCCN 2016007876 (ebook) | ISBN
9780738218717 (hardback) | ISBN 9780738218724 (ebook)
Subjects: LCSH: Weight loss—Popular works. | Nutrition—Popular works. |
Diet—Psychological aspects—Popular works. | BISAC: HEALTH & FITNESS /
Diets. | HEALTH & FITNESS / Weight Loss.
Classification: LCC RM222.2 .M526 2016 (print) | LCC RM222.2 (ebook) | DDC
613.2/5—dc23
LC record available at http://lccn.loc.gov/2016003903

First Da Capo Press edition 2016
Hardcover ISBN: 978-0-7382-1871-7
E-book ISBN: 978-0-7382-1872-4

Published by Da Capo Press
A Member of the Perseus Books Group
www.dacapopress.com

Da Capo Press books are available at special discounts for bulk purchases in the U.S. by corporations, institutions, and other organizations. For more information, please contact the Special Markets Department at the Perseus Books Group, 2300 Chestnut Street, Suite 200, Philadelphia, PA, 19103, or call (800) 810-4145, ext. 5000, or e-mail special.markets@perseusbooks.com.

10 9 8 7 6 5 4 3 2 1

To your right to
feel good without
being good.

Contents

INTRODUCTION   IX

STEP 1: EMBRACE THE FOUR NAUGHTY MANTRAS   1
Old Rule: Be good–or feel bad.
Naughty Way: Don't be good, or bad–be Naughty!

STEP 2: JOIN TEAM NAUGHTY   9
Old Rule: Start a diet.
Naughty Way: Join the thousands on my antidiet movement!

STEP 3: STOP THE SHAME GAME   21
Old Rule: Meanies and the media have power over us.
New Rule: We have power over us.

STEP 4: MAKE GUILT YOUR BITCH   39
Old Rule: I shouldn't have eaten that cookie.
Naughty Way: That cookie won't eat me up.

STEP 5: LISTEN TO YOUR BODY   57
Old Rule: You need to follow a diet plan.
Naughty Way: Let your body take the lead.

STEP 6: FIND YOUR P-SPOT   73
Old Rule: Nothing beats an orgasm.
Naughty Way: No foodgasm, no orgasm.

Contents

STEP 7: EAT NAUGHTY FOODS   89

Old Rule: Choose diet food that supports your weight loss.
Naughty Way: Choose quality food that supports your desires.
Plus: A Guide to the Top 50 Naughty Foods

STEP 8: COOK WHEN YOU WANT   119

Old Rule: 1,256, 1,257, 1,258 calories
New Rule: Count on feeling better with every bite.
Plus: 30 Naughty recipes!

STEP 9: CHILL THE EFF OUT   177

Old Rule: Downtime is for lazy people.
Naughty Way: Sleep your way to the top.

STEP 10: CHANGE YOUR BRAIN, CHANGE YOUR BODY   203

Old Rule: Exercise your willpower.
Naughty Way: Exercise your imagination.
Plus: 18 Naughty Tricks for Getting More Out of Doing Less

BONUS CHAPTER: 237
24-HOUR DAMAGE CONTROL—80 WAYS TO KICK FOOD
GUILT TO THE CURB

Notes 250

Metric Conversion Chart 263

Join Team Naughty Today! 264

Acknowledgments 265

Index 266

INTRODUCTION

*Take my hand, Naughty Girl.
I want to show you something.*

IT'S RIGHT OVER HERE: the white sandy beach of a quiet little getaway that's closer than you think.

Our little nautical nirvana is empty–just you and me and a pitcher of rum punch with fresh limes. The dunes shine porcelain under the golden sun, and the cloudless sky meets the rolling waves of the Caribbean in an uninterrupted mural of blue, with only an occasional fishing boat intruding on the horizon. This is the Naughty life. This is Mojito Beach.

And look: here comes another woman, strolling until she stops near us. She slides her sunglasses up to the top of her head and squints at us through the beams of light.

Her name is Sharon. She's got a mojito, too, and she drains the last of her plastic cup as she flops down in the sand next to us. "I'm trying to relax," she says after introducing herself, adjusting her sarong so it covers her thighs. "I have a hard time doing that." And maybe because she downed that drink too fast, Sharon tells us her story:

"My husband and I are here celebrating our fifth anniversary. Well, we're *supposed* to be celebrating. Last night, we had a whole plan to rekindle the excitement. But the only thing we rekindled was the same old fight we always have," she says. "I was feeling fat after dinner, and then I didn't feel comfortable getting naked because it was too bright. When I pulled away, he lost his patience, and then he lost . . . well, you get the picture. I waited until he fell asleep and then I raided the minifridge."

"I dunno," Sharon continues, staring out to sea, "I feel like I'm in a bad place with eating. I know what I'm *supposed* to eat, and *think* about eating right constantly, but somehow, that just makes me eat more. And then I feel this crushing guilt. I wish I could just disappear and show up on an island where I could start over–an island without anyone else to make fun of me, an island without Toblerones."

She turns to you, as if seeing you for the first time, and looks mortified. "Oh my God, this is so embarrassing! Can you even relate!?!"

Well, dear reader, I ask, raising my mojito (and an eyebrow): Can you?

I can. That was me, all day long, for years. On the surface, you wouldn't think Sharon and I had much in common–and, to be honest, you and I may seem worlds apart, too. I used to be a model from South Africa making my name in London, with the brand-name labels to prove it, and no husband to please. You'd look at me–with my Diet Coke and size 0 dress–and think I had it all together. Or at least, that's what I thought at the time. But in fact, I was also "in a bad place." I'd eat too much and then I'd make myself pay. Pay with feeling bad. Pay with restricting calories. Pay with another 1, 5, 10 miles on the treadmill. Only to give in to temptation. And hate myself for it. Again. And again. Like Sharon.

And like millions of other women today.

Just look at YouTube, where videos about body shame–by people rich and poor, young and old, like Sharon or like me–regularly get millions of views. "My name is Sadie Carroway Robertson," says one teenage reality star into her webcam, "and I wear a size 2 in a dress and eat all the time." "And I was so addicted to food," says a blond mom, in another, "that I was over 300 pounds." "What I'm confessing to is not moderation," says a thin twenty something pumping a dumbbell, in yet one more. "I was bingeing on bad food all day, every day, for months." "See, the thing is," says Sadie, "I'm telling you to share the reality of things: I struggle with jealousy, and I struggle with comparing myself to other people. I struggle with worry." "And so I had this view of myself that was *horrible*," says a brunette student.

"I *hated* the body I was in."

Comedians like Nicole Arbor don't help. Her YouTube video "Dear Fat People"–in which the slim blonde compares the overweight to slow-moving zombies–has been seen by more than 7 million people, riling critics and getting banned from YouTube temporarily. She defended it as "satire" on *The View*. But cohost Raven-Symone wasn't having it. "There's a lot of different foods out there that have ingredients in them that some people get addicted to, that they can't help the size that they are," she said, adding that she's been 180 pounds her whole adult life. "It's borderline bullying," agreed cohost Michelle Collins.

And a lot of us are bullying ourselves. Google **"body shame"** and you get **22 million** results. Try **"guilty after eating"** and you get **19 million**. And enter **"bad food day"** and up comes **358 million** links! That's 300 million more than Leonardo DiCaprio! And I personally surveyed thousands of women around America and they all said the same thing: they were sick and tired of feeling bad while trying to be good. You can see why, like Sharon, we all might long to join the Weightless Protection Program–a place where you can start over without anyone judging you, without anyone knowing your deepest, darkest food secrets. You can see why we all might need that mojito.

THE SAD TRUTH IS, there are a lot of women who suffer from serious eating disorders that doctors can diagnose and try to treat. But there are far more of us who suffer from something else–something that drives us to eat too much, diet too much, sweat too much, and worry too much. It's a full-blown eating disorder that few doctors will diagnose or treat. Its name? Food Guilt. I had it for years. You probably have it, too.

Guilt makes us want to be good.
And that's exactly why you should be Naughty.

And that's exactly why I wrote this book. The Naughty Diet says screw guilt and pass the wine. It's the antidiet diet, breaking the traditional rules of dieting–and all their man-made, media-hyped, me-focused hypocritical restrictions–so you can be free to lose weight without losing yourself. And by the end, you *will* lose weight–a psychic weight off your shoulders, shame from your brain, and extra flab from everywhere that matters.

The Naughty Diet means:

- **YOU'LL NEVER HAVE TO worry about willpower, guilt, or perilous perfectionism.**

- **YOU'LL NEVER HAVE TO feel like you let yourself down.**

- **YOU'LL NEVER HAVE TO feel bad about what you ate.**

- **YOU'LL NEVER HAVE TO fail again.**

- **AND YOU'LL BE your healthiest, happiest self ever.**

This is a nutritiously delicious eating plan for life–and a movement. And you won't be rising up alone.

Thousands of women who follow me on Facebook and Twitter have already declared themselves Naughty, freed from guilt, signing their names next to the Naughty Manifesto or sharing the Naughty Mantras online: "I agree to never let a cupcake hurt me." "It's okay to want what I want." "When in doubt, take a nap." "I do crunches. Nestlé Crunches." Thousands more signed up after an excerpt from *The Naughty Diet*, called "I Eat Slim Shamers for Breakfast," went viral on Yahoo! (Read it for yourself on page 32.) In it, I shared my lifelong experiences of being judged for being too thin, and generated nearly two thousand comments–from women large and small, and a shocking number of men, too.

"We all care about how we look to other people–in at least some small way–and that is not a bad thing," wrote one commenter. "The issue is when we let it dictate how we feel about ourselves."

"Dear Melissa," wrote another, "If you were fat, people would be nasty to you, and since you are thin, people *are* nasty to you. As long as you and your doctor know you are healthy, tell those people to go to hell."

"It's painful to try to be what society thinks is beautiful," wrote another woman. "Look at the comments. We are not alone."

This book is for them, and for you, and for Sharon. And there's a reason this has resonated with so many: the Naughty Diet bloody works, like Bloody Marys on a hangover.

How is it possible? To have your Red Velvet and eat it, too?

Because this book will—and this is where the heavens part and the trumpets blare—*change your entire approach to food.* You'll learn how to stop obsessing about calories, master your cravings, revamp your approach to exercise, and banish negative thoughts before and after eating. Get outside your head, woman! Then I'll give you the tools you need to change *what* and how you're eating, so you can indulge intelligently, with luscious recipes and sensual pleasure. Everything is informed by a team of the country's top researchers and clinicians—I call them Team Naughty—not to mention my own research, done as a certified integrative nutrition health coach.

By the end, you'll never feel anxious about "dieting," which will free you up for what's important: living, with a healthy, sexy body; a blissful mind; and room for the indulgences you crave. Like, you know, sex.

Unlocking your feelings about food is the first step in unlocking your feelings about yourself. The Naughty Diet will get you there. Join me, join Sharon, and "Be Naughty! Not Guilty!" like the thousands of women who've already joined us on Mojito Beach. If you're reading this, congratulations Naughty Girl, you're already on your way.

Melissa

Step *1*

EMBRACE THE FOUR NAUGHTY MANTRAS

OLD RULE:
Be good–or feel bad.

NAUGHTY WAY:
Don't be good, or bad–be Naughty!

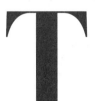HERE'S AN OLD SAYING ABOUT THE powerlessness of humanity: Man plans, God laughs.

I'd like to amend that: Woman diets, God delivers pizza. (And cookie dough ice cream. And cheeseburgers. And chocolate.)

The crux of the Naughty Diet is granting yourself permission to find pleasure when eating that pizza. It's granting yourself permission to be Naughty.

So, what exactly is Naughty?

Naughty is somewhere between "perfect" and "nasty." Nasty is what makes us fat. Nasty is revolving your entire diet around eating whatever you want whenever you want. Nasty is a supersize order of In-and-Out and falling into a food coma before sex.

And perfection is, of course, unattainable. We've tried. And trying to be perfect is what makes us feel guilty, and then go and eat something nasty.

Naughty, on the other hand, is in the peaceful center. On the Naughty Diet, the majority of your day will indeed revolve around employing (and enjoying!) the principles of healthy living, as well as healthy eating. But you'll experience them not as restrictions, but as releases. Each chapter is built around a series of Naughty Steps: science-based, life-tested, attitude-adjusted approaches to food, exercise, and life management that, far from telling you what you have to do, instead free you and let you live life to the fullest, without shame, guilt, fear, or confusion. As a result, you'll have more energy, look better, and feel strong, sexy, zippy, and zesty. But by doing so, you'll also allow for indulgences: chocolate, wine, bread, cheese. Now balanced, the guilt–and the pounds–will melt away.

Let's face it, if your body needs some calories, then dammit, your body is going to get some calories. It's going to get those calories by making you sick, by messing with your mind, by sending you craving signals. When we try to control our body and our life by controlling calories we set ourselves up not just for failure, but for true damage–physical and emotional.

FOUR CORE NAUGHTY MANTRAS

I will not count calories.

I will not make myself go hungry.

I will commit to the single best source for my food.

I will no longer feel shame.

Control, denial, failure, punishment; control, denial, failure, punishment. This is the cycle in which we live. It is not healthy. It is not fun.

And it is definitely not Naughty.

Here's why the Naughty Mantras are so important:

I Will Not Count Calories

WHEN YOU GO TO a wealthy person's home, there's one thing you don't typically see: a table piled high with hundred dollar bills on it. That's because wealthy people know that dollar bills are not the measure of wealth. They own real estate, stocks, bonds, fast cars, fine art, parts of businesses, maybe a politician or two. That's what being wealthy means. It doesn't mean having a lot of Benjamins lying around your house.

In the fight for a rich physical life, calories are like dollar bills. If you just sit around counting them all day, they're not going to be doing what you want them to do–which is to work for you. Counting calories is for chumps.

In fact, I recently came across a 2014 study in which researchers looked at 154 different countries and tried to correlate calorie intake and diabetes risk.[1] Now, you know how this plays out: people who take in more calories gain more weight and have a higher risk of diabetes. So, obviously . . .

Oh, wait. No. That's not at all what they found. When they compared the effects of adding 150 calories a day–that's about 5,475 additional tablespoons of butter a year–to a person's diet, they discovered that diabetes risk went up . . . not one bit. The number of calories people ate made zero difference. What actually matters is where the calories come from. When they looked again, but this time at people who got their additional 150 calories from sugary soda, risk skyrocketed by 700 percent!

In another study with the not-so-subtle title "How Calorie-Focused Thinking About Obesity and Related Diseases May Mislead and Harm Public Health," the researchers explain that the problem with eating low-calorie food is that you're also getting low-nutrient food.[2] You're not getting a solid return on your investment.

And yet 72 percent of the women I surveyed said calorie intake affects whether you think you've had a "good" or "bad" day, and a third of them admitted they count calories to feel "in control." Don't you get it? You're sitting around, counting dollar bills, while everyone else is getting fabulously rich.

I Will Not Make Myself Go Hungry

TAKING A BREAK FROM eating works. A little hunger can be a good thing.

But I'm not concerned about the occasional cleanse or fast–both of which can be nourishing for body and soul. I'm talking about the extreme, self-punishing type of food restriction that so many of us engage in from time to time.

In a 2014 study, Swedish and Spanish researchers put men on a diet of 360 calories a day (that's about 3 ½ apples) and made them exercise for nearly nine hours a day for four days.[3] The men lost an average of 11 pounds. But the majority of the weight they lost wasn't fat, it was muscle. And that's a great recipe for gaining back even more fat. Muscle–not the big, hulking kind, but the kind that gives you long, lean legs and sleek obliques–also burns fat. Lose it through constantly starving yourself, and over time, you'll set yourself up for even more weight gain.

I Will Commit to the Single Best Source of Food

AS A CHILD IN SOUTH AFRICA, I grew up with the food you would call healthy and "real"–unlike in America in the 1980s, our foods hadn't yet begun to be manipulated with chemicals. We didn't have corn syrup or MSG in everything. On the rare occasions I did encounter additives like high-fructose corn syrup? I went nuts for it! I even arranged playdates with a girl at school whose parents offered unlimited Coke and Twizzlers! Nasty!

Later on, I dedicated myself to the pursuit of a different kind of dietary drug–artificial sweeteners. If it had "sugar-free" or "zero-calorie" on it, I'd toss it down my gullet to feed the emptiness created by my hunger and dissatisfaction. Nasty!

Little did I know, a study by Harvard researchers that looked at over 120,000 healthy women and men over the course of twenty years found that weight gain was most strongly associated with heavily processed foods as compared to "high-quality" foods of the same caloric value.[4]

In other words, nasty foods–even low- or zero-calorie foods–make you fat. Naughty foods–even those that contain plenty of fat and carbs–don't.

I Will No Longer Feel Shame

YOU CAN SEE THE CYCLE beginning to rotate, can't you? Obsess over calories. Starve yourself. Binge on junk when you can't take it anymore. Those are the first three steps in a nasty food cycle. The Fourth Horseman of the Chunkalypse isn't what you do, it's how you feel. And this is where you start to take back control. You see, here's the secret of all secrets:

You don't feel bad about yourself when you get fat. You get fat when you feel bad about yourself.

Mindf*ck!

Of course, there's a connection between emotions and weight gain. At first, I figured it was simple and obvious: feeling bad leads to eating bad. There's a whole body of science around this: In one study, two groups of female college students described as "restrictive eaters"–girls who were trying to be "good"–were invited to sample donuts.[5] (Can you imagine how bad that might make you feel afterward?) But one group was given a lesson in self-compassion first. "I hope you won't be hard on yourself," the instructor said. "Everyone in the study eats this stuff, so I don't think there's any reason to feel real bad about it." Both groups of women were then asked to taste-test candies from large bowls. Most women ate some of the donuts and candies. But researchers found those given the pep talk ate significantly less in both situations, while those who weren't given the message reported feeling guilty and ended up "emotionally" eating as a result.

But it turns out there's more to it than I thought. Yes, studies show that when you're stressed, you eat more cakes, cookies, and chips–more nasty food and fewer Naughty foods.[6] But something even more devious happens: When you feel bad about yourself, your body raises its levels of a stress hormone called cortisol. Cortisol behaves like the bad guys in those *Taken* movies: It kidnaps all your blood sugar and holds it captive in a dungeon (in this case, deep in your belly, in the form of visceral fat). Once your blood sugar is low, hunger hits, and you get all Liam Neeson: "I have a very particular set of skills." (I can use the GrubHub app.) "I will find you." (And order you with extra cheese and a side of garlic bread.) "And I will kill you." (Gobble you up.)

The bottom line: Stop counting every calorie and logging every food you eat. Instead, embrace the good foods of the world, push the nasty ones away, and, at times, go ahead and stray. Pretty simple, isn't it? Eat good foods, which will help you forget bad foods. And get Naughty as needed. But it isn't simple. Because we're preconditioned to live by the rules. To get Naughty, you have to change your entire approach to food. You have to let go, eat with the flow, and reclaim your mojo.

That's what I'm here to help you do!

The Naughty Girl Manifesto!

Pull up your skinny jeans, throw on some killer heels, BYOB, and repeat these mantras after me:

We quit dieting.

We eat what we like. And sometimes we like dessert.

We count compliments, not calories.

If it makes us feel good, it's good.

We ban food bans.

And food intolerances are intolerable (without a doctor's note).

Our (wine) glasses are always half full.

Chocolate is a superfood.

We sometimes take our medicine in vino form.

We sometimes drink alone.

But we're no bloody Bridget Jones.

We don't give up when we give in.

We know that it's never too late to turn
things around.

We forgive, forget, and take a nap.

When in doubt, we take a bath.

We will not be defined by our weight, who we date,
or what we ate.

We dress to impress—ourselves.

We abstain from abstinence.

We moderate moderation.

We eat "emotionally" with love and passion.

We are quality freaks, not health freaks!

Pleasure-seeking is our MO.

We are food lovers. And amazing lovers.

We have many guilty pleasures.
(And we're not telling.)

Regrets? What regrets?

We know what we want. And get it. Because we like
who we are. Finally. It's that easy for us.

And we're sorry/not sorry: We're Naughty.

JOIN
TEAM NAUGHTY

OLD RULE:
Start a diet.

NAUGHTY WAY:
Join the thousands on my antidiet movement!

I will not feel guilty for seeking out the things
that make me feel good. #NaughtyTweet

I WASN'T always Naughty.

For most of my life, I was a classic Good Girl–exactly the kind of girl I was brought up to be, exactly the kind of girl most of us are brought up to be. I wanted to do everything the "right" way, so that I would fit in, win approval, and find love. And yet all along, I felt as though the women I admired–the ones who looked effortlessly slim and seriously stylish, and who enjoyed rich and exciting lives–had some sort of secret that I wasn't privy to. The harder I tried to be one of "them," the more helpless and hapless I felt.

If I had a lowest moment, it happened several years ago at a casting in London. As I sat in a long, sterile hallway that afternoon, peeling a banana–the only food I'd been allowing myself during daylight hours–another model passed by and snipped, "Do you know how many calories are in a banana?"

Calories? I had no idea!

"A lot!" she scoffed.

Taken aback, I wondered, *What can I "safely" eat?* Suddenly fruit, what I thought was an innocent food, became dangerous. Because it had "calories."

And calories weren't safe in my Skinny World.

From that point on, I started to measure all food in calories.

High calorie = very bad.

Low calorie = bad.

Zero calorie = perfect!

That's when my food issues really began.

I became an expert at ignoring my hunger cues, hoping they'd just march on by. There were days when I managed to get from sunrise to sunset on sugar-free gum, sugar-free lozenges, and sugar-free soda. I spent my hours thinking about *not* eating. ("No calories. Perfect!") I was good. I was in control. I was safe.

But I wasn't. People who are in control don't self-punish. People who are in control don't see discomfort and denial as "victories." Life isn't a Tough Mudder competition, and there's no award for "Most Oppressed Woman," no matter how hard so many of us seem to work to win it.

In fact, what I thought was control was the exact opposite. By the time I got home at night, I was so irritable, ravenous, and empty that I'd do anything to fill that void–the saltier, sweeter, fattier, nastier, the better. That was, of course, until my Aha moment.

The Naughty Aha Moment

AHA MOMENT, the precise instant when your sad, old, restricted life ends and your new, guilt-free, Naughty life begins.

IF YOU WANT TO PICK up some really bad habits, try hanging out with models.

Early in my career, I shared an apartment in Milan with an international coalition of unhealthy obsessives. There was the Romanian chain-smoker who lit up in bed upon waking and last thing at night. Her only sustenance throughout the day: sugar-free Red Bull, espresso shots, and a few blocks of cheap white chocolate. Svetlana, the sixteen-year-old Lithuanian, was on a "grape diet"–nothing but grapes and "fat-burning" ice water for her. I recall once walking in on her slowly and almost shamefully eating a pink yogurt, with a baby teaspoon and baby appetite. Our defunct '50s fridge could easily have passed for a piece of modern installation art.

When I got back to London, I sank deeper into this desperate cycle–one that accelerated after the banana-shame. Every single day was an exercise in self-denial, and most nights all resistance crumbled. I went to bed disappointed in myself, pledging to try harder the next day. *Tomorrow, I'll be good.* As a result, I was skinny fat–thin but hardly strong and healthy–sallow looking and shallow thinking. (After all, how can you have an intelligent dinner conversation when you're focused on figuring out the carb count in an artichoke?) I looked miserable, because I was miserable.

SKINNY FAT, in which the female form appears thin, but upon closer inspection has little muscle tone or strength and is soft to the touch.

THE TURNING POINT came many summers ago in the South of France. Although I was a seasoned traveler with a sparkly social life in London, my first trip to St. Tropez, and Le Club 55, blew me away. I'd been invited to lunch–a meal I invariably tried to skip–and expected nothing more than a quick bite of salad and Perrier.

Yet what I saw around me, under a canopy of overgrown bamboo, were beautiful people, young and old, indulging unapologetically. The rich hum of movie stars, aristocrats, music moguls, and billionaires alike stimulated all my senses. I couldn't believe the sight of the glamorous Joan Collins, in all-white linen, red lips, and a big sunhat, dunking chunks of bruschetta into olive oil. A few tables away, Jay Z, Beyoncé, and Bono tucked into burgers and steak frites like nobody's bidness. Amidst the A-listers were rich, perfectly coiffed, perma-tanned Frenchmen on their third bombshell wife and third glass of Ott rosé! The well-heeled patrons were all chic, de rigueur thin, and casually-passionately eating and drinking whatever they fancied, in this lavish diet-free enclave.

I was seduced.

I, too, wanted to toss back big rich hair, with big wines and rich entrées, completely carefree. So I agreed to allow myself the freedom to eat whatever I truly desired for breakfast, lunch, dinner, and in between. I said yes to croissants, caviar, heavy canapés, fine wines, foie gras, gelato, steak tartare, Bellinis, beef filet, bread and butter, olive oil dressings, sea bass, spaghetti alle vongole and decadent desserts. Club 55 showed me how food and wine can be celebrated *sans le guilt* and with full enjoyment. In the words of Edith Piaf: *Non, je ne regrette rien. No, I regret nothing!* Each and every mouthful of that holiday was memorable. Finally, I stopped looking at food in terms of good/bad, fatty/low-fat, scary/safe, and healthy/unhealthy. And I stopped counting calories. It was simply food, and the tastier the better and the richer, well, the less I needed, naturally.

I was listening to my body and navigating the restaurant tables guilt free and pleasure full. Best of all, the only thing I gained that holiday was a naughty nonchalance toward food (plus a pricey penchant for foie gras!) I remember picking up a little jar of truffled foie gras and an assortment of crackers at Hédiard in the Nice airport for my flight home. I was free. Freeeeee at last!

FRESH BACK FROM FRANCE, I threw myself into research, enrolled in Nutrition School, and tried to understand the allure of the jet-set who could celebrate life and look great.

And the magic part was this: Once I unlocked the Naughty secret, my

INDULGE INTELLIGENTLY, find gratification in quality foods you're passionate about—instead of Pecan Pie Pringles.

skin started to glow, my perennially low mood lightened up, and my body woke up and got healthier. Instead of being "skinny fat" I started to tone up. I didn't gain weight. Instead, what I gained was vitality, strength, and the verve to live well and eat well. And as I shared it with my friends, they signed on, too, and began to see that this plan was working for them, as well.

But could we eat cookies, ice cream, candy, and chips at all hours? Of course not. That's Nasty, gal. But what we could eat was rich, delicious food—where and when we wanted. All we had to do was learn to listen to our body—and understand when it wanted us to be good, and when it wanted us—no, needed us—to be Naughty. The kind of Naughty that's too good to regret.

That luscious lunch was my Aha moment. Your Aha moment is now—*right now*—wherever you're at—St. Tropez or Santa Fe—size 2 or 20. The Naughty Diet is you saying you've had enough with your life until today. Everything before this sentence is the old you. Everything after is the new you, the Naughty you, an empowered you. Welcome to the club!

HAVING SPENT SO MUCH TIME around models and fashionistas, I just assumed that food issues were endemic to my social circle, shared again and again like a Grumpy Cat video gone viral. We were all struggling to be thinner, more glamorous and more fabulous. We put so much pressure on ourselves and exerted so much effort to appear effortless.

But as I've traveled and made friends with people from all walks of life, I've learned that Food Guilt is no more rampant in the techno clubs of Berlin or the oldest members' clubs of London than it is at the county fairs of Fairfield or in the hair salons of Harrisburg. And that's what inspired me to start the Naughty Diet, and develop my own principles for living well and loving life. Nowadays, whenever I run into friends I haven't seen for a while, they always ask me the same question. And I always give them the same answer. And it became so common, I just had to start a Twitter account and spread the wisdom:

"Wow, you look amazing! What's your secret?"
Oh I just lost all that Guilt. #NaughtyTweet

Flashing that Naughty attitude got such a huge reception, I realized there was a whole world of women just like me, waiting for someone to stand up and say, "Enough! Enough with the guilt, enough with the dieting, enough with letting men, the media meanies and my own warped thoughts make me feel bad." I started a Facebook page, too:

You wouldn't let a disrespectful asshole live in your house.
Why would you let one live in your head?
#NoMoreFoodGuilt #NaughtyTweet

Within days I had hundreds of women liking, favoriting, sharing, and commenting on my Naughty musings about Food Guilt, Fear, and Shame. And the healing power of Pleasure, too. Within months the Naughty community had grown by the thousands.

I met women like Monica, age 36, from Des Moines: 30 pounds from the voluptuous size 12 at which she felt sexiest, and addicted to diet food and calorie-counting. And Emilie, 24, from Culver City: a natural size 2 who didn't need to diet but who still subsisted on black coffee and salads because her relationship with her boyfriend was always on tenterhooks. And Janet, 44, from Tampa, who never ate sweets in front of her husband, but who sneaked cupcakes behind his back and then punished her sweet tooth with hours and hours of cardio. And on, and on—hundreds of women from all over the world—women of different dress sizes, with different food preferences, and varying health and weight goals. But what we all shared was a pleasure-seeking spirit that was fed up with being bullied, put down, and shackled by Guilt. What we all shared was a desire to be who we are inside.

We all wanted to be #Naughty.

As my social media following grew, I realized I needed a way of collecting all the stories and feedback I was receiving and collecting it in one clear, authoritative place. I sent out an invitation for women to take a survey, and share more of their thoughts and feelings about food, diets, and body image.

More than ten thousand women responded, and the stories they shared made me more determined than ever to bring the Naughty Manifesto to the world.

Here's what I discovered:

More than 80 percent of women feel guilty after a decadent restaurant meal; and nearly the same number of women said post-dinner sex would be completely off the menu.

Nearly 50 percent have dieted down a dress size(s) to appease a man; and another 25 percent would consider it if pressed.

Among the single ladies who took the survey, **70 percent** believe their body size was the reason for their relationship status; and **more than 80 percent** of women feel a hotter body would improve their sex life.

In addition, **70 percent** of women practice restrictive eating habits the day of a dinner date.

And it's not just romantic relationships that take a hit; **more than 50 percent** of women admitted to canceling or wanting to cancel plans with a girlfriend on a "fat day."

But this one depressed me the most: When **given the choice to be happier, smarter, or thinner, the majority of women chose thinness as the Holy Grail.**

And when I asked these women what Food Guilt meant to them, I got Food Guilt Poetry:

Inevitable

Pointless

Part of the Deal

Overeating

Overwhelming

Overrated

Always There

Every Day

Everywhere

Exhausting

Chocolate (x359 Guilty girls)

Huge

Buzzkill

Scales

My Enemy (Scary!)

Powerful

And my favorite: Dumb!

What struck me–what made me so damn angry–wasn't the fact that we've all experienced Fifty Shades of Guilt, but that we're so accepting of it. "My Enemy." "Always There." "Inevitable."

Really?

Imagine being told a computer virus had infiltrated your online banking account and was draining away your life savings. Or that a parasite had poisoned your drinking water and was ruining your family's health. Or that a rival was making a play for your man behind your back.

Meh. Inevitable . . . What are you gonna do? Gotta live with it, right?

Not bloody likely! You'd be a woman on fire, and no one would stand in your way when it came to fixing the problem, saving the day, and holding on to what's rightfully yours. The bankers would be ducking for cover, the doctors would be racing against the clock, and that would-be paramour would be tied up inside somebody's trunk. Am I right?

Yet Food Guilt is as damaging to your physical, financial, and romantic health as any malware, any bug, any backstabbing homewrecker. And most of us just accept it. *My Enemy . . . Always There . . . Inevitable.*

Well, no. It's not. It's time to grab Food Guilt by the scruff of the neck, give it a few slaps across the cheek, and kick that bitch to the curb. It's time to get Naughty.

Joining Team Naughty

I'm in control, out of control, but never under control.
#NaughtyTweet

MY NAUGHTY SOCIAL CHANNELS were ablaze. The poll was packed with shocking revelations. And everyone I spoke to about the Naughty Diet told me, "You have to spread the word. There are so many women out there wrestling with this, and no one is talking about it."

But I couldn't do it alone. I needed people who understood the female mind and the female body, and how the two work together to help–or harm– our weight-loss goals. I needed a Vice Squad. I needed a Down & Dirty Dozen. I needed Comrades in Charms.

I needed Team Naughty.

My first call was to one of the biggest medical rule breakers I know: Tasneem Bahtia, MD, who has all the training of a traditional Western medical doctor, and none of the restraints or prejudices. Few people have such a high degree of training and influence in medicine and still talk about spirit, the mind-body connection, and the ways in which traditional Eastern medicine can soothe and heal just as well as the pill or the injection. You just do not get straight talk from most docs the way you do from Dr. Taz.

But more importantly, Taz has been there. She's spent time under the thumb of Food Guilt, and she's wrestled it to the ground and dug a stiletto heel into its throat. When I told her about what I was doing, she hopped on board with the same enthusiasm I have when someone offers me a glass of wine.

"Food is the one thing women can control," she told me. "You can't control how much money you make, you can't control the behavior of the people around you. But the one thing you can control, supposedly, is what you put in your mouth. So, it's a sign of failure when you can't control 100 percent the one thing you're supposed to be in charge of. If you fail at that, you're going to fail at everything."

Then Taz opened up about her own struggles with Food Guilt:

"I'll be honest, I have come a long way myself. I went through a period of time in medical school when I tried to control everything I put in my mouth.

Medical school is a time when you can't control anything, including your schedule. It's intensely stressful. There was a group of girls I hung out with who tried to gain control through food. A couple of them were anorexic, and I learned from them how to turn controlling food into a game. I weighed less than I ever have, and I didn't realize what I was doing to myself until I started to see the cosmetic changes—my hair was literally falling out. I got sick, and then I had to get better. And that's been part of my food journey."

So, how did she get over it?

"Nowadays I realize that food gives me everything—it gives me pleasure, it gives me energy, it determines the way I look. But it doesn't determine the way I feel about myself. I've had to learn to have the proper relationship with food. Honestly, I don't beat myself up any more. But that comes from establishing a strong sense of self-esteem, being healthy and happy in the work that I do and the relationships that I have."

She continued, saying, "The first thing is to set realistic expectations. We all overindulge. That's human nature. But I set the expectation that if you can eat healthy 80 percent of the time, then you're fine."

Another expert whose advice I trust is Heather Quinlan, PhD. She's a psychotherapist, but not just any therapist. She specializes in self-image, and when I say the words *Food Guilt*, you can almost hear her eyes roll on the other end of the phone.

"There is something warped about the way women talk to one another," she told me. "It's the whole idea of 'fat talk': 'Oh my thighs are so fat!' 'No, they're not! Look at my belly. I'm Jabba the Hutt.' 'Ugh, I ate so much at lunch.' 'No, you're fine; I shouldn't have had the cookie!' It almost becomes a competition to prove which of us is the most shameful."

Listening to Heather reminded me of my days spent playing the food and body "shame game" against the toughest rival of all—myself.

She went on to explain the difference between Food Guilt and Food Shame. Guilt is about regretting something we *did*. Shame is when it becomes personal: I did this thing, so I'm a bad person. It's about who we are: our character. And when we create strict rules about what we eat, and then break those rules, well, we're shameful. We're bad. If I love Oreos, and if I make myself a rule that "you can't have Oreos," then if I have ONE Oreo, by definition I've lost control because I've broken the rule. And now I'm bad.

I don't want to be bad.

But dammit, I don't want to be good, either.

I just want to be Naughty. Follow me and I'll show you how.

STOP THE SHAME GAME

OLD RULE:
Meanies and the media have power over us.

NEW RULE:
We have power over us.

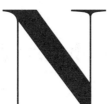

EW YORK: at a sun-drenched bistro table, the brunch-time light dancing off their crystal glasses, three girl-friends dressed in white unfold a cloth napkin onto their lap and prepare for a mimosa-fueled gossip fest.

Houston: In the corner of a wood-paneled sports bar, redolent of stale beer and hot wings, a gaggle of women eye the pool table, appreciating the fit of a pair of jeans on a long-haired boy who looks just like Brad Pitt in his *Thelma & Louise* days.

Las Vegas: On the faux-leather couch of a nightclub, their blouses glowing pink and green under the spinning lights, three ladies struggle to be heard over the throbbing bass of their favorite DJ.

It could be Ibiza or Indianapolis; Dublin or Des Moines; Athens, Greece, or Athens, Georgia. The place doesn't matter. The language doesn't matter. Neither do the faces and names of the women involved. Wherever women gather together, the conversation is likely the same.

"She's not fooling anyone with that shirt. If she got any more muffin top they'd have to call her Cornbread."

"Seriously, those thighs are so skinny, how does she stand up? She's like an ostrich."

"Did you see those arms jiggle? What's her blood type, con queso?"

Put a group of us together, and we so often turn into an attack squadron. We fly in formation, set our sights on an enemy target, and we fire away.

But in the end, every mission becomes a suicide mission.

"Oh, my arms jiggle worse than that! They're so flabby!"

"No, they're not! Look at mine! Total handbags!"

Our self-esteem is constantly under the gun, and not just from the forces around us. We love to compare ourselves to others, to see where we fall in the hierarchy of body shape, to inflict maximum damage on the competition. But of all the injuries to our ego, the worst are the ones that are self-inflicted.

This chapter is a call for a ceasefire.

Don't Judge, Judy

I RECENTLY TOOK a blank notebook to a country club in the Hamptons for a rosé-infused afternoon of writing and research. There I overheard a group of women having lunch on the patio near the tennis courts. They were eyeing a group of female club members engaged in a game of doubles.

"Joanne doesn't look on top of her game," one of them said.

Another chimed in, "Yeah, quite unfortunate. She's looking sloppy this week. But look at Danielle. She looks awesome. Best I've seen her."

"I heard she went to some 'retreat' and came back totally transformed and refreshed . . . if you know what I mean," said another.

"Oh my God. Seriously? She'll be back to square one in a month's time. Guarantee it. Quick fixes are so lazy and never work."

"I know, right? So, what are we getting for lunch, chopped salad?"

Then I realized: it wasn't the women's tennis skills they were critiquing, but their looks.

I was reminded of Ashley Judd's "puffy face" interview on NBC's *Rock Center*, when she felt compelled to respond, poignantly, to accusations that she had gotten cosmetic work and was hiding it.[1] Her puffy face was, in fact, the result of a medical condition, she said, pleading for the onslaught of negative comments to end.

And of Giuliana Rancic, who was viciously slim-shamed by women online for using a surrogate mom, reportedly because she worried about pregnancy weight. One female Instagrammer went so far as to say she was "setting a bad example for other women."[2] The truth: she had breast cancer and was taking medication, so couldn't carry a child.

And of Adele, and Hillary Clinton, and Carrie Fisher, and Kate Middleton—all criticized, not for their performance, but for their appearance.

And I thought about a conversation I had with my own bestie, over dinner a few nights earlier. We'd each changed at least six times before meeting, and finally decided on baggy pants and loose tees that did nothing for our slim, healthy figures. We both admitted to our fear of being judged for looking too old, too try-hard, too fat, or too thin in anything remotely "sexy." This was a casual dinner with my best girlfriend!

When I dug into the research I discovered feeling pressure from fellow females to look a certain way isn't just a thirty-something epidemic. A recent study found that among teenage girls, peer competition—not television or social media use—was the strongest predictor of a negative body image in the short term and eating disorders in the long term.[3]

And another survey that canvassed thousands of women ranging in age from sixteen to seventy years found that "fat talk"—the self-degrading "if you're fat, I'm huge!" conversation that has become somewhat of a social ritual among women—was common across all ages and all body sizes.[4]

So, what the hell is going on in the minds of women today? Why are we so quick to judge ourselves and our fellow sisters?

Are we all just a bunch of hardwired mean girls?

On Wednesdays We Wear Pink

I REACHED OUT via the Naughty Survey, to see just what was happening with us all, and found that across America,

Nearly two thirds of women say they have been body-shamed by another woman for being too fat or too thin. And **nearly 50 percent** of all women admit to having consciously body-shamed another woman for her looks.

Nearly 70 percent of women feel pressure from female friends to be thinner or "the thinnest"–**more than double** the number of women who admitted to feeling pressure from men to lose weight or be thin.

More than 95 percent of women admit they're more judgmental of other women's appearances than they are of men's.

And when I asked the source of a negative body image, "other women" proved to be the culprit–more than **three times as influential** as men, and **twice as responsible** as the media.

This went against every supposition I'd made going into this project, and against every "women's studies" class I'd ever taken. Aren't we women the victims of an oppressive, sexist society ruled by the patriarchy?

Are we really doing all of this to ourselves?

I needed to draw on the expertise of Team Naughty.

I got on the phone with Dr. Alexandra Corning, director of the Body Image and Eating Disorder Laboratory at the University of Notre Dame. I shared my survey results, and asked her the burning question: Are we women eating ourselves alive?

"Melissa, this is about women and social comparison," she said.

All humans have an innate desire to evaluate their own success. We do this with everything, from grades to salaries. And appearances, too. But unlike hard dollars or solid scores, there's no objective, definitive measuring stick that tells us how close or how far we are from a beautiful, desirable body ideal. Sure, there are images in the windows of Victoria's Secret, but they don't represent our real lives or our social circles; those women aren't our competition. Comparing our curves to Miranda Kerr's gives us no more information than comparing our IQ to Einstein's. The only way we can truly judge ourselves and our place in the pecking order is to constantly measure how we look versus the other women in our lives. Consider:

Only 30 percent of women say they would like to look like those women featured in magazines.

A whopping 80 percent disagree with the statement that "celebrities and models are an important source of information about body and beauty ideals."

"We all have a tendency to compare, and it's not necessarily a bad thing," said Dr. Corning. "Social comparison can be a positive motivator for self-improvement. But what's going on with women right now–what is problematic–is *what* we're chronically comparing."

"It's not a part of our DNA to run around comparing our bodies and our diets to other women," she continues. "It's because we're constantly bombarded with messages from the media that suggest we should; that beauty is the center of the universe. What I've found particularly interesting in my research is that women who express symptoms of eating disorders tend to be chronic comparers. Almost everybody has found that people who struggle with disordered eating consistently have lower self-esteem. So, if you're already struggling with body image or engaging in restrictive eating, you're probably, statistically speaking, more prone to compare yourself to other women. It becomes this vicious bidirectional downward spiral: the more you compare, the more you diet; the more you diet, the more you compare."

CHRONIC COMPARERS, Women stuck in what Dr. Alexandra calls "a vicious bidirectional downward spiral: the more you compare, the more you diet; the more you diet, the more you compare."

OFTEN, WOMEN COMPETE in ways that are wildly self-destructive. The standard of beauty we all rail about isn't set by men or the media, but by *us*. It's a way to reduce the competition for mates, according to Joyce Benenson, a researcher at Emmanuel College in Boston.[5] We demand a status quo, then punish those who openly try to attain more than others–shaming the slender, debasing the beautiful. If a new hottie shows up in the office or at the bar, the other women in attendance may unconsciously do whatever they can to undermine her, hoping to force her out of the circle–and decrease their own odds with the men in the gene pool.

Go back to that brunch table, that sports bar, that Vegas club. Judging others, comparing ourselves to them, criticizing our own body–it's become a driving part of how we socialize with one another. It's like that "on Wednesdays we wear pink" scene in the movie *Mean Girls*.

And we take it home with us. It's not like we leave it at the bar.

More than half of the women I surveyed said they'd "gone hungry" because they felt shamed for their size; **55 percent** started a diet immediately; **42 percent** canceled their social plans. And a sadder-than-The Notebook-sad **46 percent** said they "quietly wept and felt more shame!"

Even worse, **70 percent** of respondents said they felt shame every single day–with **22 percent** admitting they feel it "constantly, every minute."

Yet how many of these women "fought back and felt proud" when body-shamed? **Only 26 percent.**

But . . .

We're not victims. We're in control. We can stop ourselves from falling under the wheel; we can break the wheel.

"Think about childhood," said Dr. Corning. "You're climbing a tree. You're not thinking about whether your shorts still look good on you from that angle on the ground. You're just climbing a tree. That could be our existence. Wouldn't it be lovely? We could mow our lawns and walk our dogs and do our jobs and not have to look hot. We could just exist. We can have that, but we have to stop talking about beauty all the time."

Language Is a Virus

THAT DOESN'T MEAN IT'S EASY. Our social conditioning, our subconscious mind, and our ingrained need to identify our place on the totem pole conspire to make comparisons a driving force in our lives. The first person I called was Dr. Andrea Meltzer, a social psychologist at Southern Methodist University.

"From an evolutionary perspective, and even on a biological level, heterosexual women have a strong drive to reproduce," says Dr. Meltzer.

I reached out to her because of an amazing piece of research she'd published, in which she followed a group of women who were trying to manage their weight, and discovered that the days on which they cut the most calories also happened to be the days when they were at peak ovulation.[6]

"Why would that be the case?" asks Dr. Meltzer. "Well, social norms tell us that 'thinner' is more desirable to a mate and that restricting calories can get us there." That's the smoking gun: hard evidence that we instinctively try to make ourselves thinner whenever we feel the biological urge to hook up. And yet that terrible pursuit–to be thinner, more attractive, to climb higher on the social totem pole–is making our daily lives miserable.

"What my research shows is that women with a positive body image are happier in intimate relationships–that's independent of body size. Not only are they happier, but their partners are happier too," Dr. Meltzer says. "It suggests, hey, if you feel good about yourself, it's going to extend into other aspects of your life."

But how do we get there? Here's the Naughty 5-point plan:

1. **Remove the targets.** Take note of the things that are making you feel crappy about your appearance and remove them. That means if your crew spends half its time talking about how bad they all look, and the other half talking about how bad others look, well, it's time to roll with a new squad.

2. **Give yourself the thumbs-up.** Dr. Alexandra's research shows that women who practice regular self-affirmation have less body dissatisfaction and are less self-critical of their body. Write down a handful of affirmations that are balanced, a little bit sexy, and somewhat realistic. Then practice affirming yourself at least twice a day; morning and night. Keep them on your phone. Tattoo them on your body. Buy a dog and name him "Good Enough." Jot them on Post-its, buy the tee-shirt, make them your login passwords, sing them in the shower or repeat them out loud, looking yourself straight in the mirror, with a smile on your dial. It may feel silly at first, but soon these positive words will start replaying in your head and help drown out the

self-degrading talk. Practicing positive self-affirmation, consistently, will help keep you focused on being your healthiest-sexiest-happiest self.

Here are a few Naughty favorites:

I accept myself deeply and completely.

My body is uniquely beautiful.

My body is the perfect fit for me.

I am brave, strong, and important.

I am a complete masterpiece, in progress.

I do enough. I am enough.

I'm not afraid of mistakes, because I make decisions from my heart.

The food I choose to eat or not eat does not make me good or bad.

I regret nothing, because I do the best I can.

I am exactly where I am meant to be.

I will not feel guilty for seeking out the things that make me feel good.

I will be at least as good to myself as I am to everyone else.

I am in control, because I know how to let go.

Good enough is good enough.

I am good.

I am enough.

3. Shut up! Dr. Alexandra put it best: "People don't realize there's this thing called self-regulating. It's a nice way to say 'shut up!' Just because a thought pops into your head, does not mean you should say it." Misery may love company, but by sharing your own low self-esteem thoughts, you're just spreading them. In fact, research has proven that fat-talk is contagious. It's the body-shame equivalent of yawning.

4. Find your healthy-sexy. For years I grilled my family members, challenged doctor friends, obsessively weighed myself, studied medical charts, and prodded boyfriends for insight as to what I needed to change about my body in order to be more attractive. Do I need to gain weight? Lose fat? Build muscle and where? Stay the same? Is it okay I weigh this much? How much did you weigh at my age? Did I look better then or now? Honestly. Tell me the truth.

That was until I discovered the naughtiest news of all: My body had the answers to all these questions. I just needed to throw out the damn scale with others' opinions—let go and listen. That's because my body—like yours—runs on healthy-sexy cruise control known as "set point." The theory purports your body uses genetics, hormones, hunger cues, and behavioral changes to defend a 10- to 20-pound weight range at which it feels and looks its very best.

When you go below or above your body's natural set point,[7] both appetite and fat-burning adjust to try to return you to a healthy, sexy, comfortable weight range. Drop too low and your metabolism slows to prevent you from starving; gain a wee bit too much over the holidays and fat-burning speeds up . . . slightly. Unfortunately, the body defends against weight loss more than weight gain, which is why it's easier to put on weight than lose it.

Individual set points vary. One woman with a petite frame may have a set point range between 110 and 120 pounds, while another woman, same height, may be healthiest at 130 to 150 pounds. Bottom line: Your set point is uniquely yours, and it's a range, not a fixed number. It's totally normal and healthy to have a closet full of varying dress sizes. So, forget about weight charts, and for goodness' sake, stop comparing your own healthy-sexy to hers!

Whether you're a natural size 10 to 12 dying to be a size 4, or a whippet-thin size 0 to 2 who would kill to be a curvy size 8, don't let this theory upset you. "Set point" is the biggest dysphemism in the history of medical science. It should be termed, and I suggest you correct anyone who utters the theory henceforth, "healthy sexy range." Because that's really what it is: Not only will you be able to eat (and drink!) the foods you love at this weight without fear of bingeing or ballooning, but you'll LOOK your best. (Yes, even if it means gaining a few pounds–I actually look and feel my fittest at the higher end of my naturally low set point.)

Not to mention you'll be able to sleep soundly, perform better at work, laugh more often, have a healthier sex drive, and just be an overall happier, more dazzling, and charming version of you. No shame in that game.

5. **Change the conversation.** Ignoring body-shaming or fat-talking–or worse yet, participating–doesn't help to break the pattern. It can be scary to stand up to friends. But pull up your big-girl skinny jeans and do it for Team Naughty. Acknowledge the situation and change the conversation. You don't have to be aggressive, or start talking about current affairs. However, something simple like "Hey, let's not be mean girls" or "Come on, you don't need to hate on yourself to get a compliment from me. [Insert genuine compliment here]" can subtly diffuse an otherwise damaging, pointless discussion about looks. Then talk about something far more fun like, uh, men, love and sex!

Here are a few more choice words, from those who took my Naughty survey, when asked what they'd tell women who body shame others.

Most ladies were compassionate:

"Let's hold each other up, not put each other down."

"Don't judge. You don't know her story."

"You are causing more damage than you can imagine."

"Don't we have it hard enough without attacking each other!?"

Some were confrontational:

"Don't you have anything better to do with your time?"

"I might be fat but you're dumb. I can lose weight, you won't gain brain."

"'Fuck you.' I know, that's not mature, but it's my standard response after all these years."

But one woman spoke for all:

"If we continue to do this to each other," she wrote, "there is no hope."

Fact is, men will always make stupid from-Mars comments. Marketers will always airbrush the bejesus out of even the most beautiful women. And even the best plastic surgeon in the world can't turn us into Gisele lookalikes (even Gisele's not happy being Gisele, if you believe the plastic surgery rumors).

But what we can control are the words that are coming out of our own mouth. As Laurie Anderson said, "Language is a virus." When we question out loud whether our own body is good enough, we may well cause other women to do the same. And when we judge other women for their appearance, we feed the very culture that makes it OK to value women based on their looks.

I Eat Slim–Shamers for Breakfast

HERE'S THE ESSAY I WROTE for Yahoo! that broke the Internet.[8] I braced myself to be shamed for writing an essay about shame but, in fact, of the nearly two thousand comments, *none* were from trolls–instead, men and women alike shared their own scarring stories. I've included some of my favorite comments at the end.

You and I haven't met yet, but if we are ever introduced one day, here are some of the conclusions about me that you'll jump to before our handshake even ends:

- I'm narcissistic.

- I'm a control freak.

- I hate myself.

- I'm not very bright.

- I suffer from an eating disorder.

- Oh, and . . . you'd better ease up on the handshake, or you might break me!

You'll embrace one or more of these assumptions because the very first thing you'll notice about me–before my green eyes, my South African accent, my smile, or my hopefully gracious greeting–is my body shape.

See, I'm skinny. Too skinny, apparently.

Before you roll your eyes and tell me how lucky I am to have this "problem," heh-heh, hear me out: I'm one of an increasingly wide array of women who are judged for being too lean–from Taylor Swift to Kendall Jenner, Angelina Jolie and Bethenny Frankel, who recently made headlines for posting an Instagram of herself wearing her 4-year-old daughter's PJs–she's been fighting off accusations of anorexia ever since. And earlier this year, Giuliana Rancic was slim-shamed online for supposedly using a surrogate because she didn't want to gain pregnancy weight. The truth: She was grappling with breast cancer and taking medication that prevented her from carrying a child.

Taking shots at a woman for being "too skinny" is the last safe bastion for haters. People who struggle with obesity still battle stereotyping, but it's no longer socially acceptable to make harsh, judgmental comments about a person's heft. We've outgrown the idea that a woman's being "too heavy" is entirely her fault—or even that a few extra pounds isn't something that many men, and women, can admire (thank you, Meghan Trainor).

But being too thin? Oh, that's definitely my fault. And there's not a whisper of social approbation about mentioning it, either to my face, or behind my back. Not only is it socially acceptable to say hurtful things; most people who do don't even register that their comments might have a negative impact. ("Look at you! You're so skinny!") Body image expert Heather Quinlan, C.S.W., explains that "shamers may think nothing of their hurtful comments—maybe because society sometimes teaches that you can never be too rich or too thin." How could anyone feel badly about calling me "too thin"? But it's an insult in the form of a compliment, what Quinlan calls "an underlying resentment toward people who appear to be effortlessly thin." That's me; The Skinny Bitch.

Making negative assumptions based on a person's weight is never healthy. Overweight or thin, it sends the same damaging message: Your body does not conform. And body image is a sensitive subject for nearly every woman who does not look like Adriana Lima naked. According to DoSomething.org, approximately 91 percent of women are unhappy with their bodies. Being thin doesn't make me any different.

Growing up, and even into my late teens, I never thought about being too slender. But as I've progressed through my 20s, my self-consciousness has grown. The fact is, putting on weight—healthy weight, that is—just isn't easy. Like my mother, sister, grandmother, great-grandmother, and great-great grandmother, I am genetically slim. Like green eyes and high cholesterol, slim runs in my family.

And naturally thin women suffer the same food guilt, ugly days, fat days or "I hate my thighs" moments. I'm as insecure about my stick-thin arms as the next woman is about her thick arms. When we shame any female body, we shame the collective female body. Body positivity only flourishes in the absence of body-shaming—no matter what form. Suggesting the salad to the heavy-set girl hurts her, no matter how well-intentioned; bombarding me with snide asides, back-handed compliments, unsolicited concern and advice, the skinny sarcasm, bad jokes, negative body speculations, unfair accusations, unwelcomed weight policing, and annoying food-pushing has the same effect.

Recently, I posted a photo to Facebook that elicited a great example of how clueless most of us are to these feelings. First, a male friend commented with what he thought was a compliment:

- *"You put on a little weight! looks lovely."* **Ouch!**

- **A female friend of a friend quickly chimed in:**
  *"Hey, whoever said you've put on weight is crazy–
  you're a rail!"* **Ouch again!**

Two comments, both intended to be compliments, both landing their arrows right at the heart of my body issues.

If I seem overly sensitive, that's because I am!

See, I don't really worry about my weight until someone else decides to. That's when I feel obliged to explain that: Yes, I eat. No, I don't live in the gym. Yes, I am healthy. No, I'm not a health freak! Yes, I do love food. No, I don't take drugs. Yes, I am small but it's a matter of genetics and metabolism. No, I do not throw up. Yes, I had breakfast! No, I don't eat just salads. Yes, I am happy. Yes, really happy. No, I'm not overdoing it. Yes, I have always been this size. No, No, No . . . Yes, yes, yes!

These days, I'm really most ashamed for feeling ashamed. I've wasted too many good years feeling slim-shamed–of letting my body image be negatively impacted by others' negativity. I've donned shoulder-pads and horizontal stripes. Given up running, forced down muscle-bulking protein shakes (revolting) and even lied about my weight–adding at least five pounds, if you're rude enough to ask.

So what motivates slim-shaming? Is it ignorance, envy, thoughtlessness, malice, real concern, tough love, or bitter resentment? Perhaps it's a benign misunderstanding of body type: naturally thin? Regardless of the reasons and influences at play, I now know that this sometimes "too thin" (for some) body of mine is who I am.

An "Anaconda" ass ain't my DNA. No matter your size, reaching total body acceptance requires all that "self love work."

And body-shaming sure sets a woman back.

Reprinted with permission from Yahoo!

Of the 1,800+ comments on the Yahoo! piece, here are those that struck a nerve among other commenters, and me . . .

IDLF

There are always going to be a-hole haters out there. Women are CONSTANTLY shamed for being too overweight, but when they measure up to Barbie doll standards, they are also derided. If you think it's bad being a woman, try being a man who is naturally thin. Men are all supposed to look like G.I. Joe. Be yourself and be proud of who you are.

MONTIE

I was once compared to a refugee from a Nazi Concentration Camp. Being Jewish on my mother's side, with the knowledge that some of their family were murdered in Europe; let's just say that comment didn't go well for all concerned. If you don't like someone for their size or shape, fine; but why act like you've never advanced past a grade school mentality? It just shows who the smaller person really is.

NO NAME

New rule, you meet a person and they are a bit chubby you say "nice to meet you!" and if you meet someone who is skinny you say "nice to meet you!" Let's all treat people as people and let people handle their own problems.

AMANDA

The only place where anyone makes overtly negative or backhanded comments [about me being thin] is in the Midwest, when I go back to visit my family in my little hometown. I stick out like a sore thumb there, and people aren't used to seeing people that look like me. It can be a bit awkward, but it's never been that big of a deal. I just challenge them to an eating contest and then move on.

ANONYMOUS

I have endured this kind of treatment my entire 40+ year life. I have been accused of being a drug user for 30+ years, "randomly" selected for drug testing on the job an average of 5 times a year out of a staff of 13 (other co-workers seem to have that test done with their annual physical). I do not recall a single week in my life that some random person has not been compelled to make some off the cuff remark or waitress singling me out about being able to have dessert without guilt. No matter how you try to brush it off or discuss genetics, the same die is always cast and it does cause deep emotional scarring over the years.

KATHRIN

Thank you for bringing to light the fact that "Thin" and "Sick" are not the same thing.

And I love this comment from a dude named ERIK, who took my intro and flipped it:

You and I haven't met, but if we are ever introduced one day, here are some of the conclusions about me that you'll jump to before our handshake even ends:

• I'm lazy.

• I have no self control.

• I hate myself.

• I'm not very bright.

• I don't exercise.

• I'm a slob.

You'll make at least one of the assumptions before I even greet you. All because I am overweight.

Anybody can say pretty much the same thing. Every group has its stereotypes that are not always based on truth. Might be nice if people stopped judging other people based on their appearance.

And finally, I had to share this one, from a guy named RON . . .

I have been married to my best friend for 10 years now, She is 6' at 114 pounds. To say the least she is very thin and always has been. I don't think there is a single comment that she hasn't heard—she was targeted as a child because of her size. I have even on occasion stepped in to correct the words of people who think it's ok to make negative comments on the matter of her size. My wife eats more than any other human I've ever known and still can't gain a pound. I see the looks she gets, I hear the comments that they say and it just #$%$ me off if I'm honest.

The fact of the matter is she is just a skinny woman, and to be honest the only thing I would ever change about her is simply the way she sees herself. I wish every day that she could see herself thru my eyes, see the beautiful woman that she is. I have given my life to the most incredible and beautiful woman I have ever known and she is perfect in every way. Be proud, ladies, of your body and of who you are—anyone that tries to conform you to what they think is beauty is just a true jackass.

Step *4*

MAKE GUILT YOUR BITCH

OLD RULE:
I shouldn't have eaten that cookie.

NAUGHTY WAY:
That cookie won't eat me up.

I regret nothing, because I do the best I can.
#NaughtyTweet

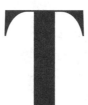

HE MORE I READ UP about food guilt and shame, the more I discovered that there's a whole body of research around it. Yet I have read dozens of books about diet, fitness, and nutrition—and in not one single one of them does the idea of guilt come into play. Oh, I know lots of "facts" about weight loss . . .

- **FACT:** Reducing food intake by 200 calories a day will result in an annual weight loss of 20.857 pounds (20.9 on leap years).

- FACT: There are ten times more fat cells in the average American's belly than there are dollars in Donald Trump's bank account (and he's worth $4 billion!).

- FACT: LeBron James's digestive tract is 67 feet long. (Yours is ten times your height, too.)

BUT AS NAUGHTY BOY Stephen Colbert once said, "Facts matter not at all. Perception is everything." You can put a fact out in the wilderness alone, and it will starve and die. Out of context, they mean nothing. Especially when you put them up against what I call "Truths."

- TRUTH: Women feel guilt far more intensely than men do. (A research team at the University of the Basque Country in Spain actually came up with a way of measuring guilt, and it found the same thing.)[1]

- TRUTH: When we feel guilty about food, we can't lose weight. (A study in the journal *Appetite* actually found that women who associated chocolate cake with guilty feelings were less successful at losing weight than those who associated it with celebration.)[2]

- TRUTH: When we feel guilty about not losing weight, we overeat and gain more weight. (In fact, a study in the journal *Psychological Science* found that those who felt shame about breaking rules were more likely to break them again.)[3]

MY NAUGHTY SURVEY proved that most of us can't handle the truth. And by most, I mean most: **95 percent of women** said they feel "bad" after indulging, with **45 percent** revealing they almost "always" feel that way. Let that sink in. Of 10,000 people surveyed, 8,800 said they feel guilty much of the time, and will likely break the "rules" again. We're in a prison system, with pink fluffy handcuffs–and the system's broken.

How ladies dealt with that guilt was equally revealing: **81 percent** said they'd make sure their next meal was "good" and cleansing. A sizable **45 percent** said they'd go one step further and skip the next meal altogether. And **61 percent** said they'd make up for it with more exercise–longer, harder, faster. This isn't balance. This is compensation. And compensation is an award paid to someone who's been injured! And who's injuring you? You! It's time to bust free. It's time for The Lambshank Redemption.

What Is Food Guilt Exactly?

I KNEW WHO TO ASK FIRST, my Naughty sister-in-arms, Elise Museles. Elise is a certified eating psychology and nutrition expert based in the Washington, DC, area, and runs the blog "Kale & Chocolate" (best name ever!), a site devoted to living a deliciously healthy life. She's helped thousands of people deal with their Food Guilt–and has first-hand experience in battling her own.

"I grew up in Los Angeles and went to an all-girls school, so you can imagine the pressure I imposed upon myself to seek perfection with food," she says. "It wasn't just me–finding the perfect diet was pervasive. So I lived with a lot of 'clean eating' rules. I studied voraciously, read every book on the shelves and tried every diet under the sun. And each time I took a bite, I thought: Is this food approved? What would this expert say or that one?"

She called her affliction "eating perfectionism"–the opposite of Naughty.

"I never had an eating disorder, but this was disordered eating," she remembers. "I was tense, uncomfortable, and it was impacting other parts of my life. I beat myself up all the time."

Years later, she became a successful attorney, downing kale salads and green smoothies like a super good girl. "But I realized I wasn't fully nourishing myself," she says. When she met her mentor, Marc David, author of *The Slow-Down Diet*, a book about mindful eating, Elise had an epiphany–her Aha Moment. "What you think is just as important as what you eat" she says. "I was eating clean but I was destroying the nutrients with stress! So I started to think of my food choices as individual choices–not ones dictated by diets–and that took the pressure off. It was life-changing."

Elise quit law and devoted her life to helping others "get their green on, and their chocolate, too." She describes Food Guilt as "harboring any negative feelings about the choices we make about what to eat... or not eat."

"It can be a passing thought," she says. "Like: 'I shouldn't have eaten that.' Or in more extreme cases, we make it a moral judgment about ourselves: 'I'm so "bad"' turns into a 'bad' feeling that goes way beyond a food choice–it impacts your entire self-esteem."

This snowball effect may make some emotional sense, but look at it logically and you'll quickly reveal Food Guilt's weakness. "First of all, there's no morality with food!" says Elise. "There are smart choices or better choices, but it's not 'good' or 'bad.'"

Willow Jarosh couldn't agree more. The registered dietician founded C&J Nutrition with Stephanie Clarke, RD, and together, they've devoted their practice to debunking food's power.

"No food is good or bad," they told me. "Sure, they can make us feel less or more energized or we can eat too little or too much and cause discomfort...but the food itself doesn't have the power to be good or bad or make us good or bad by eating association."

Unfortunately, that doesn't stop us from falling victim to it–and often at the worst times–when our reserves are running low. Think of Sharon on Mojito Beach on her anniversary. Or, "Just look at the survey you did," says Elise, "where women said they wouldn't have sex after indulging in a decadent meal. It goes back to self-love. You can't love someone else until you love yourself. Food Guilt permeates your psyche."

How to Make It Your Bitch

AS ELISE AND I TALKED, she sketched out the steps she takes her clients through, and shared them exclusively with me, to share with you. It's a short-but-sweet series of questions to ask yourself:

Why am I feeling this guilt?

What can it teach me?

How can I release it?

What's my action plan for moving forward?

LET'S GO through them one by one.

Why am I feeling this guilt?

"When we have these emotions, they're there to teach us something," says Elise. She told me about a client who felt guilty every time she ate–you won't believe this–bananas. Specifically bananas. (Maybe it was that model friend, from long ago!!!) "She'd tell me, 'I can't drink that smoothie,'" remembers

Elise. "But she ate other foods with natural sugars in it. There was something about the banana. During our sessions, we discovered that 15 years ago, when she went on the Atkins Diet, one of the 'bad' foods was bananas, because it was higher glycemic. Meanwhile, my client felt comfortable eating dates. Her Food Guilt was not rational!"

Elise calls this thinking "judgements attached to food because of outdated beliefs." It could be something from your childhood, or a formative experience in your twenties, or maybe just an offhand comment by someone important to you, made during a vulnerable moment. Once you identify the source, ask yourself, Do I even really feel that way anymore? After all, you change your fashions, month to month, or decade to decade; you can change your feelings, too.

"When people realize where some of this unwanted behavior comes from—whether it's binge eating or being consumed with guilt—or how they got into this cycle in the first place, it releases some of the anxiety. When you can see the origins and make sense of the 'why,' you'll feel less shame about your behavior."

What can it teach me?

When Elise's client realized how irrational she was being, she was able to get past the banana thing. Elise has had other clients who realized their guilt associated with certain foods was not just mental, but physical, too. "You could be feeling bad about pizza because it doesn't agree with you," she says. "The guilt may not even be about having the pizza. It might be that it doesn't feel good in your system, so then you can dig deeper and see if maybe you're gluten intolerant or dairy doesn't work for you. If you get behind the why, it can uncover some of those truths."

How can I release it?

Elise has an expression I love: "Healthy eating is a journey." Did you eat one cookie too many, in your opinion? "You don't have to wait for the New Year or tomorrow to get back on track—you have the power to move forward with your healthy behaviors at any time," she says. "It's not about punishment. It's releasing it—saying, OK guilt, you taught me this lesson, but I'm going to get back to treating my body with respect."

Willow and Stephanie also believe being nice is key to being Naughty. "Change your language," they say. "We work with clients to speak to themselves with kindness and understanding. And we discourage using the terms 'good food' and 'bad food' but instead have them put food into the context of how it makes them feel, energy-wise and fullness-wise. For instance, a cupcake is neither good nor bad–but if you aren't hungry and aren't in the mood for sweets, eating a cupcake might make you feel sluggish and overly full. It wouldn't be the best choice for you at that time."

What's my action plan for moving forward?

The book you're holding in your hands is a good start. *The Naughty Diet* is devoted to changing your entire approach to food. Elise also recommends something simple: Think about your next 24 hours, and look forward to them. "When you say, 'I'm going out to dinner and going to have dessert,' then you get comfortable with it," she says. "When you say, I'm going to spin class the next day and making myself a green smoothie–not as a punishment, but because it makes me feel good–there's something to that, also. I am a huge proponent that we can build in and give ourselves permission to have these indulgences and then move on. That releases the power they have over us."

To Elise's terrific list of questions, I'll add one more: **What does my body want?** The next chapter is devoted to just that–turn down the noise and listen to yourself, and watch Guilt wilt. "A lot of the issues we face with Food Guilt have to do with the messages we're given by society," agrees Elise. "There's Paleo one day, veganism the other, and people just don't know what to do, so they follow all these diets and restrictive eating patterns. But what that does is take you *outside* your body.

"If we all listened to our bodies," she says, "there'd be a lot less Food Guilt."

Seventeen Shades of Toxic Food Guilt

Guilt comes in many forms. Which of these do you relate to most?

1. Ethical Food Guilt: caused by eating veal (animal cruelty), foie gras, non-free-range poultry products, white shark soup, or any other endangered species.

2. Extravagant Food Guilt: caused by eating très, très chère foods. Those white truffles and beluga were how much? Make sure there's a willing and able Black Card at the table.

3. Mindless Food Guilt: caused by mindlessly eating your way out of boredom, stress, disappointment, low mood, frustration, guilt! (Yes, I have felt guilty for eating out of guilt! Double bugger!)

4. Sore Food Guilt: caused by eating for any of these physical reasons: periods, jetlag, hangover, etc.

5. Procrastination Food Guilt: caused by doing food, instead of doing x. Just think back to your college years . . . filled with all those "study (snack) breaks."

6. Dark Food Guilt: caused by abusing food for the sake of abusing yourself. More reckless than a random binge due to the explicit intent to eat till you're sick. Followed by an overdose of guilt.

7. Processed Food Guilt: caused by not eating fresh, real foods. When the only fresh thing you've had all day is the sprig of parsley atop a microwave lasagna.

8. Lazy Food Guilt: caused by snacking on packaged crap instead of washing, peeling, chopping, and preparing something fresh and gorgeous from the fridge.

9. Numbered Food Guilt: caused by obsessively calorie-counting, weighing yourself (and food), dress-size dreaming. Stress × 100 to the 1 billionth power.

10. Sugar Food Guilt: caused by eating dessert (dieters don't do that!) combined with a sugar crash.

11. Drunk Food Guilt: caused by a drunk binge, usually late-night, home alone, with fatty, high-calorie (or still frozen) foods. Frequently occurs post blah date. Instead, brush your teeth and grab your vibrator as soon as you get home.

12. Recovery Food Guilt: caused by spending an entire day(s) nursing a hangover or heartbreak with food (and possibly, probably more booze) as medicine.

13. TV Dinner Food Guilt: caused by not making a meal out of mealtime—i.e., not plating your food and instead eating off whatever flat surface is closest to Netflix. Siblings include: Standing and eating, walking and eating, eating in the car . . .

14. Food-Pusher Food Guilt: caused by overeating to appease a body-shamer. Leaves you feeling guilty AND pissed off!

15. OTT Food Guilt: caused by a totally over-the-top restaurant meal or an unbalanced day(s) of eating, like cheese and wine only, for an entire weekend! Or week . . .

16. Gone-Green Food Guilt: caused by buying super green juices, bunches of kale, and multiple heads of lettuce and watching them rot in your fridge. Good intentions, though.

17. Restrictive Food Guilt: caused by undereating, meal-skipping, overexercising, purging, or any other restrictive eating behavior. You are being a Meanie to your body, and you know it.

No matter which type/s of Food Guilt we suffer from, to be truly Naughty, we need to find a way to let go of the guilt, give up the idea of total control, and relax about food, so we can start indulging ourselves, enjoying the food we love, and love the way we look and feel.

Here's three ways to start:

- **SHRED YOUR THOUGHTS.** The next time you catch yourself red-handed—or orange-handed, with an empty bag of Doritos—and you feel Guilt bubbling up . . . Freeze. Grab a pencil and a piece of paper, or a cheap eyeliner and a napkin, and write down exactly how you feel. "I'm bad. I broke the rules. I feel nasty." Now—and this is the important part—rip that piece of paper to shreds as if it were an old Valentine from your toxic ex and toss it in the garbage. What worries you masters you. Don't let Food Guilt rule you. Remember: YOU are at the top of the food chain.

- **EVACUATE THE ZONE.** Now, immediately leave wherever you are. Seriously, even if it's on a terrace overlooking Lake Como, and Clooney's there, and he's whispering in your ear about how Amal and he are having a rough patch, and his breath is like sugar blossom tickling the nape of your neck . . . leave. Ciao! Don't linger at the dinner table, calculating how many calories you've just consumed; don't hide under the covers afraid to see how many empty bags of drunken late-night snack foods you may find in the kitchen. Remove yourself from the location, and change your mindset.

- **DO SOMETHING DIFFERENT.** Once you're in a new location, do something new to distract yourself. Go for a walk outside. Get a manicure. Be old-school cool and go to the library and read a book. If you want to sit at a coffee shop and write a love letter to George, do it. The most important thing is that you distract yourself and move on to something new.

That's the short-term plan for politely dismissing Guilt and getting your Naughty back. But if you really want to conquer the bastard and seize your mojo, then pour a glass of wine, and take this quiz to see how Guilty you really are. And then shimmy on to Chapter 5 to learn how changing your approach to food changes everything. Think: Julia Roberts in *Eat Pray Love* feasting on pizza after stating:

I'm so tired of saying no, and waking up
in the morning and recalling everything I ate
the day before—counting every calorie I consumed
so I know exactly how much
self-loathing to take into the shower.
I'm going for it. I have no interest in being obese,
I'm just through with the guilt.

#NaughtyGirl

Naughty Quiz
How Guilty Are You?

Answer these ten questions, choose the answer that best reflects you, and then find my verdict—and Naughty Rx—for making Guilt your bitch.

1. You skip dinner, meet the girls for drinks out, and get home late—pooped and ravenous. Too tipsy to put a real snack together, you hit the Cheetos hard. The next morning, the couch is a crime scene of orange crumbs. Your reaction is?

   (a) You don't give the chips a second thought, preferring to replay how much fun you were last night. (3)

   (b) You clean up and make yourself a healthy smoothie. You make a mental note to avoid drinking on an empty stomach next time, though you know you will. (2)

   (c) "I'm such a loser! I can't believe I ate all that junk last night. I feel so gross." (1)

2. You and your partner go out for a rich Italian dinner. You over-order, overeat, and leave feeling stuffed and unsexy. At home in bed, he starts to kiss your neck and initiate sex. What do you do?

   (a) You might be feeling like a beached whale but that doesn't mean he can't pleasure you before you pass out. (3)

   (b) You turn him down with a passionate good-night kiss and say you're just sleepy and want to cuddle. He has no idea how that creamy linguine killed your mojo. (2)

   (c) Tenderly push him away and explain that's it's not him, it's you—it's *you* who feels like stuffed tortellini. You never want to hurt his feelings. (1)

3. You have a special date tonight and learn your man has booked a table for three at your favorite restaurant, to give you two more space and privacy to luxuriate. How do you justify this?

(a) Score. Because small tables? You just don't "do" them. (3)

(b) You feel uncomfortable and guilty throughout dinner—the restaurant is bustling, and your waiter keeps asking after the phantom third guest. (1)

(c) You make an exception for this special occasion and validate the bigger table by going straight for the reserve wines and tipping generously. (2)

4. You and your girlfriend have plans to grab an early bite tonight. That same morning, the guy you totally fancy the pants off asks you out to dinner. Do you . . . ?

(a) Tell him you unfortunately have plans. You can't drop your friend on the same day. (1)

(b) Immediately bail on your friend, with some lame excuse like being "bogged down with work" or feeling "ill." You and she can catch up any old time. (3)

(c) Ring your friend, explain the situation and ask how *she* feels about rescheduling. The ball is in her court. (2)

5. Your new lover is coming around for dinner. Eager to impress, you pick up food from a fine Italian restaurant. The food is such a hit that he praises your culinary skills. What do you do?

(a) Subtly change the subject, without disclosing that dinner was not your cooking. It's not a big deal—you could make this—risotto is not rocket science. (2)

(b) Bask in the glory; and pick up every brownie-point going. The way to a man's heart is through his stomach, after all. So what if you got a little "help." (3)

(c) Tell him the truth and read disappointment in his expression. This makes you regret not going the home-cooking route. You worry that he might think you're lazy/ incapable and/or not wifey or mommy material. #epicfail (1)

6. You and your girlfriend go out for drinks. Two unattractive guys start to chat you up at the bar and offer to buy a round. How do you handle it?

(a) Order two glasses of champagne and scoot. (3)

(b) Politely decline and say you have a boyfriend. You don't want to take free drinks off guys you have no interest in nor do you want to hurt their feelings. (1)

(c) Let them buy you a round and chat to them for a few minutes as a thank you. (2)

7. You ate all the cookie dough in the ice cream! What kind of gerbil are you?

(a) Guilty and sorry! (1)

(b) Sorry/Not Sorry (3)

(c) A little bit sorry . . . but it was totally worth it . . . (2)

8. Your mother-in-law insists you try her heavy noodle kugel at the family holiday party. She's practically spoon-feeding you. You . . .

(a) Eat it even though it's fattening, you hate noodles, and you're not hungry. (1)

(b) Tell a white lie: "That looks awfully delicious, but I'm not hungry—I just ate and/or had a big breakfast/lunch/dinner/etc." (2)

(c) Take the spoon, take a pretend bite, and feed it to the dog—all within view of mumsy. (3)

9. You're just a few pounds away from your LBD weight, and you have an event coming up next week. When your restaurant salad comes swimming in the dressing you specifically ordered on the side, you . . .

(a) Cry. This is exactly why you don't like giving up control. (1)

(b) Refuse the dish, and demand to speak to the manager. (3)

(c) Eat only half of the salad (delicious!) and eat a light dinner to compensate for the extra fat calories. Waste not, want not. (2)

10. You drink too much Friday and have a one-night stand with a stranger. (He looked so cute through your rosé-colored glasses!) You wake up feeling . . .

(a) Indifferent. As long as you got off. Sometimes a no-strings-attached shag is just what the doctor ordered. (3)

(b) Mortified, humiliated, traumatized—you're such a dirty slut. You're never taking your clothes off again. You race back home and spend the weekend in bed eating chocolate. (1)

(c) Disappointed that you settled for the instant-gratification, frozen-dinner equivalent of lovemaking. That's what your vibrator is for. You call your bestie who allows you to sulk over a cup of coffee, then forget about it and make fun plans to go out that night. (2)

Naughty Quiz: **Scorecard**

Score 10 to 15 points:
THE GOOD GIRL GUILTY CONSCIENCE

**The Verdict: On the charge of First Degree Guilt, we, the Jury,
find you guilty of extreme Guilt.**

You might not wear a habit and inhabit a nunnery, but you are nonetheless
plagued with God-fearing Guilt—and a senselessly big, guilty conscience.
You feel guilty about small, everyday things—from hitting "snooze" to watching
reality TV. When it comes to eating, you tend to avoid your cravings and stick
to what's "safe." You think you gain weight easily (just looking at a dessert
menu gives you bra bulge) and almost always regret indulgent treats and
restaurant meals. Is it rational? No. Does it suck? Hell, yeah!

You find it difficult to just be in the moment and enjoy yourself. You're known
to be a giver, worrier, an analyzer/over-thinker, an abstainer, perfectionist,
people-pleaser, and harsh self-critic—quick to forgive others and slow to
forgive yourself. To be frank, it's pretty darn exhausting being you.

To attain the peace and pleasure of a more worry-free and guilt-free life,
you need to start by managing your guilt more effectively and learning to feel
naughty, not bad, whenever you're a bit "bad."

Naughty is never bad. It's just a little less than good.

Score 15 to 23 points:
THE NAUGHTY CONSCIENCE

The Verdict: We, the Jury, find you not guilty of bad Guilt.

You have the ideal Naughty conscience—a moral sense of real wrong and right,
along with a healthy sense of what's nicely Naughty. You manage any guilty

feelings very efficiently and positively. You don't lose sleep (or pleasure) over some naughty behavior. Rather than wallow in guilt, you take strength from it—often using it to inspire positive actions. You learn from your mistakes. You don't delude yourself: you call a transgression a transgression and a treat a treat. But you own it, forgive it and get on with life!

For you, food is one of life's many pleasures. And oh what a pleasure it is! You know how to nourish your body and soul with a balanced, flexible diet of needs and wants—cheese and wine one day, greens and water the next. Indulgent desserts and boozy holidays may leave you with a bit of extra "fluff," but you know you can bounce right back to your healthiest, sexiest size.

You possess a logical mind, strong sense of self, and good dose of self-worth; topped with a smidgen of self-entitlement because, yeah, you know you're special. You don't feel guilty about sometimes putting yourself first.

Selfishness is seen as self-care. You think: if it makes me happy, it can't be that bad! You also know that you have to make yourself happy to make others happy. You know how to moderate when necessary and indulge when needed. When you are good you are very, very good and when you are bad you are naughty! Guilt doesn't consume you because, deep down, you know that you are a good person. Even when you feel guilty, you take solace in knowing that you are a good person who sometimes makes bad judgments. Your heart knows that you are a loving person who seeks to love and be loved. And your head knows that nobody was harmed in last night's binge.

Score 23 and Up:
THE BADASS CONSCIENCE!

The Verdict: You don't give a shite, really!

Your conscience certainly does not keep you up at night, and chances are, you wake up in the morning asking, "What do I want?" I love the spirit! But it's possible that you are quite self-centered, self-absorbed, and narcissistic, with a big ego and huge sense of entitlement, to boot. Some may describe you as tough, strong, brutally honest, and steadfast—but be sure you're not just hard, inflexible, unsympathetic, and a stubborn ass.

It's probably your way or the highway when it comes to wining, dining, and dieting. You tip only when your meal is Michelin-star quality and always make complicated alterations and requests at every restaurant meal (sometimes just to test the servers). You expect your friends and party hosts to cater to your dietary preferences if they really want you to attend social gatherings. And if not? Their loss. Your goals are more important, anyway.

You often excuse your behavior as "tough love."

But I call it a lack of empathy.

Try developing some . . . Since empathy impacts our conscience and our conscience our guilt, it is the obvious place to start. Try putting yourself in other people's shoes. A good idea is to volunteer for a charity—preferably a soup kitchen or food rescue organization—to be surrounded by people in real need. Volunteering can be sobering to your indefatigable ego that usually has no time for compassion. Just don't Instagram shots of you with orphans. #notcool

Step 5

LISTEN TO YOUR BODY

OLD RULE:
You need to follow a diet plan.

NAUGHTY WAY:
Let your body take the lead.

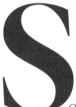

O, HOW DO YOU take control of your Food Guilt, rather than letting it guilt you?

This question popped into my head one night at a swanky jazz bar in New York City. A male model–writer friend was celebrating a just-announced book deal and invited a crew of close friends–fashion industry folk, hipsters, and a couple of trust-fund babies–to celebrate the good news. The venue was packed: filled with head-bopping, toe-tapping beautiful people sipping on mojitos. Everyone was in their element. Except for me.

The slick tap of the brush on the snare drums made me nervous; the performers were all too-cool-for-school. (Why were their eyes closed? And why the sunglasses in the dark room?) The unexpected blurt of a saxophone sounded like a mistake. It was all so random, so impromptu and unfamiliar, and so not something I could sing or dance to. "Great, isn't it!" shouted my author-slash-model mate, over a noisy piano riff that sounded to me like a hippo had plunked down on the keyboard. "How it all comes together out of chaos!"

Comes together? More like falls apart.

"I've never quite understood jazz!" I admitted.

"You're trying too hard," he said. "Stop thinking, M! Start listening. Feel the rhythm. It's not random; it's perfectly balanced. See, even the improv follows its own vocabulary and grammar. There are no rules, no right or wrong choices in jazz . . . some are just better than others."

And all of a sudden it made sense. I knew exactly what he meant.

Embrace the Chaos

FROM THE GET-GO, the Naughty Diet had one goal in mind: to give women a sensible way to escape the diet traps, the shame and the guilt, and to take back control of their own body and life. But as I began writing, I fell right into one of those diet traps myself.

See, I figured that to create a book that reached people, I'd have to do what every other diet book author has done: create a strict regimen of mealtime protocols and a buttoned-up, cookie-cutter eating plan, wrapped in scientific-sounding claims and promises—plus a blacklist of "never eat that!" food sins that every woman must eschew. Or else, fail.

But that just didn't make sense to me. Naughty girls don't like to be told what to do and when to do it (unless we're playing a late-night game of "naughty secretary"). We play by our own rules and groove to our own syncopated rhythm—a rhythm punctuated by spontaneous parties, last-minute dates, inspired workouts, and impromptu travel plans.

How could I recommend a clockwork meal plan—even one that was centered on pleasure, fun, and carbs—when I couldn't possibly follow such a plan myself? Let alone choose to. I'd figured out a pattern of eating that worked brilliantly not only for me, but for so many other women who tried it. But it wasn't a strict, traditional "diet plan," and it wouldn't be tamed by any set of prefab rules.

That's when I decided to get on the phone with Nina Savelle-Rocklin, PsyD, a psychoanalyst who specializes in food, weight, and body image issues. And Dr. Nina told me exactly what to do: Stop trying to do something exactly.

"Fact is, Melissa, 'strict and calculated' simply doesn't work. We're not robots. We're bodies, with real wants and needs that are constantly evolving," Nina said. "When you stop telling your body what it needs, and start letting your body tell *you* what it wants–you come face to face with the 'chaos' or 'uncertainty' of real hunger. That can be scary.

"But healthy, balanced, normal eating IS chaotic," she continues. "It's overindulging at times, and it's underindulging at times. It's grazing throughout the day, or it's three balanced meals. It's leaving dessert on your plate because you can have it tomorrow, or it's having a few cookies straight from the oven right now, because they're fresh. It's this trust of the internal world that people lose sight of and that we need to reacquaint ourselves with."

That was it! I had been trying to squeeze my insights and research about nutrition into a formulaic composition, when what it really needed was some free jazz: rhythm, harmony, flexibility, and spontaneity. What seems like the chaos of our body is in fact a clockwork of precise chemical and hormonal rhythms–the timing of which are critical for survival. Your heartbeat, breathing, sleep cycle, menstrual cycle, metabolism, and digestion are all rhythms that play a constant song that is health and life.

Unless, of course, you disrupt your body's natural balance with a "plan."

The Naughty Genius Within

HERE'S A RIDDLE: What do army sergeants, prison wardens, and diet book authors have in common? They all tell you what to eat, when to eat, and then force you to spend time in "the yard." Yet real life isn't like prison or the military (unless you're actually in prison or the military). And unless that diet book author is going to come to your house and blow a whistle in your ear, you need something else to keep your food life on the right path.

Fortunately, that something else is already inside you.

There's a brain in your digestive tract that holds the answers to meal timing and portion control. It's called the enteric nervous system (ENS). Get acquainted with your ENS, and every meal's like wining and dining with your own personal nutritionist. You'll know what and how much to eat, and exactly when you can afford to indulge again–without gaining an ounce.

The ENS is a complex network of 100 million neurons and chemicals that lives in your digestive tract–it's what you might call your "belly-brain." It senses and controls digestive events by sending messages to the head-brain–things like "I'd love another slice of bread," or "That's enough bread for me, thanks"–along a superhighway called the vagus nerve. Even more fascinating, studies show that in the partnership between the two body parts, your belly actually sends more messages to your brain than your brain sends back. It's like your belly is Simon, and your head is Garfunkel.

Naughty Activity
CHECK YOUR HEALTHY/SEXY RANGE

I know how it is. You can be feeling really good about yourself, jump on the scale and–dun, dun, dun, dunnnnn . . . NO! What?!? Cue neurotic behavior: reset scale, change the battery, pee, take off jewelry, check pockets for coins, remove clothes, shave legs, sit in a sauna for an hour, schedule a haircut . . . All to fudge a silly number that can't measure healthy or sexy.

And if you're weighing yourself on a Monday morning, you're only setting yourself up for disappointment. Because you probably DID gain weight over the weekend. We all do. And then we lose it again during the week, according to a recent study in the journal *Obesity Facts* that studied humans' natural weight fluctuations over the course of the seven-day week. According to the researchers, weight loss occurs in cycles. Almost everyone experiences a higher weight after weekends and a decrease in body weight during the week-days, reaching the lowest point on Friday, when we're running on fumes.

Accept the fact that weight fluctuations are normal and not necessarily a sign of weight gain. And get rid of the damn scale! Weigh-ins are for wrestlers.

The Rhythm of Hunger

SO, IF OUR BELLY is this deeply intuitive, Zen-like genius just brimming with knowledge, why do most of us do such a terrible job of heeding it? In part, it's because we're all like little puppies, constantly distracted by the next shiny thing. Living in the savannah, chasing antelope meat, left us plenty of time for quiet contemplation; today we can barely swallow the next bite of crème brûlée before our phone pings with some exciting new distraction. (And our digestive system was built for calm, not for craziness; it's the vagus nerve, not the Vegas nerve!)

But it's also because we've been taught, as Dr. Nina says, to fear the chaos of our own feelings. A "good" girl is always in control; she never gets too

And to be perfectly frank, nobody cares about that number but you. Here are seven Naughty ways to check you're in a healthy-sexy range instead:

1. Can you wriggle into jeans from the dryer without popping a button or a seam?

2. Does your bra fit? Specifically, the band size.
   (No harm if the cups have miraculously filled up.)

3. Do you have a healthy libido?

4. Do "the painters" come in on schedule?

5. Is it hard for you to recall the last time you called in sick (because you were actually sick, not playing hooky)?

6. Do you cry only for good reasons, like when you spill wine?

7. Are your hunger levels pretty stable (PMS aside)?

angry, sad, horny, lonely, tipsy, frustrated–or hungry. Instead, embrace uncomfortability and trust your gut, Girl, and get out more.

You could eat something different for lunch every single day of your life, and still not experience every mouthwatering flavor the world has to offer. So, why don't you explore more? I can guess a few reasons–sorry/not sorry for pointing the finger:

You're a Creature of Habit

WE ALL ARE. My question is, eww, who'd want to be a creature? You're human! One thing that separates us from animals is this very naughty concept, coined in a Harvard study, called a "promiscuous combination of ideas." It allows the mingling of different concepts "such as art, sex, space, causality, and friendship thereby generating new laws, social relationships and technologies." In other words, we can think. Naughtily! Do so when it comes to food!

You're Conditioned

IT'S A CLASS THING, it's a how-you-grew-up-thing, it's a product-of-your-time thing–your decisions aren't your own, they're the product of circumstance and childhood. You eat how you always ate. But wake up, McFly–you're, what, twenty something? Mid-thirties? Live not just *for* the now, but in the now. You can't blame your parents' divorce for eating bad cheese.

You're Nostalgic

THIS IS DIFFERENT from being conditioned. Here, I'm thinking of the grown-ass men who scarf down a bowl of Cinnamon Toast Crunch every morning, because they want to feel like a kid, or the women who serve Shake 'N Bake to their family because it's comforting. American food is a security blanket. But we're smothered in it. Enjoy Little Debbie once in a while, if you must, but don't invite her in the house.

You're a Control Freak

MAKES SENSE. In an uncontrollable world, we can control what we eat, because we have to cook it or buy it. But there's a reason no one has written *The Anal*

Chef. Cooking can be messy and playful and spontaneous and stimulating. And I'm not asking you to give up control. I'm asking you to direct yourself (because you're so good at it!) toward new options, maybe ones that involve spilling some red sauce. You can always lick it up.

You're on a Diet

THE FIRST THING that diet books will tell us to do: strip away the emotional attachment toward food. If you like that plan, more power to you: eat your bland old chicken breasts with steamed vegetables or kill your sense of taste with Lean Cuisines, and go on your merry way. Let's see how long that lasts. (Oh, wait, you have.) Next!

Finally, You're Just Not That into Food

HOW SAD FOR YOU, but there's hope yet. I have a girlfriend who was really passionate about Broadway musicals, the *Khaleesi*, her job, and her boyfriend–but she wasn't that into food. She described mealtimes as an annoying game of Whack-a-Mole: Bop one down and another pops up four hours later. That's admirably utilitarian but hardly romantic. If you're not that into food, maybe you haven't found the right food yet. She fell in love with olive oils and never looked back.

SET THE TABLE FOR PLEASURE

We lose something very important when we strip away our emotions from food altogether. Here's how to get your mojo up and running again:

FEAST YOUR EYES FIRST We eat with our eyes first, so presentation is essential. Always plate your food elegantly and set the table with cutlery, napkins (with napkin rings for bonus points), place mats, condiments in condiment dishes (no Heinz bottles please), and flowers or candles whenever possible. You're unlikely to pig out when you set the table for an elegant experience.

SLOWER, DEEPER, LONGER Yes, I am still talking about food! We can all agree that a great meal is an enormously pleasurable experience. By slowing down and savoring the tastes, textures, and entire moment with all your senses, you can prolong and deepen the pleasure–think of it as tantric eating. You wouldn't rush mind-blowing sex, wish your vacation would fly by or watch the season premiere of *Jessica Jones* on fast-forward, right? I rest my knife and fork.

INDULGE PASSIONATELY I used to be too afraid to get really *into* food. I avoided cooking, the Food Network, gourmet delis, and ordered just *whatev* at some of the world's finest restaurants. Oh sacrilege! Waiters may just as well have been speaking gibberish while reciting the day's specials because I was too busy counting the calorie cost. Like a jilted, burned lover, I felt totally vulnerable around good-looking food. I feared falling head over heels in love with it all. And God forbid I turned into a–shudder–"foodie"! Surely I'd get hooked on the "wrong" foods–the carbs and butter–lose all control and let myself go.

Oh, how wrong I was. See, indulging with passion puts you in touch with all your senses and this heightens the pleasure of the entire eating experience. In a fully conscious, multisensory state we never overeat–we taste, savor, and make love to every memorable morsel. A passionate eater a.k.a. gourmet/foodie/gourmand/connoisseur/hedonist/gastronome/bon viveur/bon vivant (see, I'm equally passionate about my thesaurus)–Naughty Girl eats with all she has and extracts infinite pleasure in the quality of the whole dining experience. There's no space for self-sabotage and feelings of guilt or deprivation in passionate and loving relationships–including your relationship with food.

Making food a hobby turns it into a personal, special-interests pursuit. That elevates it to new levels, high above calorie counts, convenience, and cost. Here's how:

Getting Started

- Explore one particular ethnic cuisine.

- Order unusual spices online.

- Drive to a new neighborhood specifically for a single ingredient. Today, you have more knowledge and more resources and nothing is off limits, so why not tuck in and taste some variety?

- Take a wine class; then research pairings.

- Take a cheese class; then research cheese and wine pairings.

- Take a cooking class and master 2-3 dishes.

- Where in the world would you like to go today? Eat that destination. Book Thai or Japanese, or even learn to make chicken tikka if India tickles your fancy.

- Get geeky: Learn how foods work chemically.

- Become discerning. Feel something. *Be a food snob!*

And remember: Inside you is an insatiable wild child, a hungry, feral intelligence that won't abide by anyone's "rules." To tap the knowledge of your glorious, all-knowing belly-brain, you need to train yourself to listen. Here are some clear signals that your gut may be sending you.

BELLY-BRAIN MESSAGE #1
You're craving something creamy.
Translation: You need a warm hug, not a warm mug.

Recurring cravings for particular types of food can be a sign of nonphysical hunger. A desire for ice cream or hot chocolate can really be an emotional craving for comfort and soothing.

BELLY-BRAIN MESSAGE #2
You can't find your keys.

Translation: You need a nice plate of pasta.

Your head-brain is like a picky five-year-old. It wants simple sugars, and when it doesn't get them, it gets cranky and undisciplined. That's because your brain runs on glucose sent to it by your belly-brain. One study found that just twenty-eight days on a low-carb, low-cal diet negatively impacted memory among subjects.[1]

BELLY-BRAIN MESSAGE #3
You just ate and you're hungry again.

Translation: You need a bite of dark chocolate.

A balanced meal should cover all of the four basic tastes: sweet, sour, salty, and bitter. It's this last, bitter, that triggers the hormone ghrelin, the "belly full" hormone. It's why we can eat a full sleeve of Pringles and still be raring to go. Leafy greens carry bitter flavors, as does coffee and dark chocolate.

BELLY-BRAIN MESSAGE #4
You're pissed and you want a Snickers bar, now.

Translation: You're going too long between meals.

Research shows that "hanger" attacks—the nasty combination of hunger and anger—are brought on not by hunger per se, but by low blood sugar. A shortage of blood sugar makes the brain more susceptible to frustration and less able to control impulses. One study found that having low blood sugar levels made people more likely to want to stick needles in voodoo dolls resembling their romantic partners.[2]

BELLY-BRAIN MESSAGE #5
You finished off your fries and now you've started in on his . . .

Translation: You're addicted, but it's not love.

In a recent study, researchers at the University of Michigan found that French fries were the number one most difficult food to stop noshing on once you've started. In part, that's because of their addictive combination of fat, salt, and carbs.[3] But it's also because bulky foods like French fries and pasta help relieve feelings of loneliness. They literally "fill the void," says Dr. Nina. If you find yourself constantly overeating carbs at dinner, you might need a new dining companion.

BELLY-BRAIN MESSAGE #6
You're hungry midmorning or midafternoon.

Translation: You're probably thirsty.

A study in the journal *Physiology & Behavior* suggests that 60 percent of the time we respond to thirst, it's by eating, instead of drinking.[4] If you haven't had any water after a long night's slumber, or after several hours at the office, dehydration is probably catching up to you. Quick test: is your pee yellow? Drink.

BELLY-BRAIN MESSAGE #7
Your belly rumbles

Translation: Don't mind me, all's good.

A growling stomach is nothing more than a bout of hiccups under your navel. It can occur at any time (usually in an important meeting or on a first date!), on an empty stomach or a full one, and no, you needn't respond.

BELLY-BRAIN MESSAGE #8
You can't sleep.

Translation: Let's have eggs for breakfast.

Whether you're stressed out or just jet-lagged, disrupted sleep can do a number on your circadian rhythms. Researchers say protein for breakfast—followed by carbs in the evening—can help rejigger a wacky biological clock.[5]

Naughty Activity
RATE YOUR HUNGER

Whenever you sit down to eat, you want to be hungry but not ravenous. Before every meal,* ask yourself: How hungry am I? What can I eat that will bring me the most pleasure right now? What nutrients does my body need in this moment? Allow your mind to be silent and trust your gut. The answers will emerge. Don't censor them. If you're worried your bod will be very Naughty and tell you to "order the fried mozzarella," don't worry. You and your gut have been wrong many times before and you're still here. Trial and error is how evolution works.

Aim to eat when you're at a 1 (i.e., physically hungry) and quit around a comfortably satisfied 3, with the exception of exceptions.

*Naughty Tip

Rate your hunger before or halfway through your first cocktail. Trying to gauge your hunger when you're too "relaxed" makes it one hundred times more likely you'll also "relax" your judgment as to when, what, and how much to eat as well.

The Hunger Games Scale

0. Famished. "I must eat now!" Hunger pangs. Salivating. Loss of concentration, energy, and focus. Hallucinatory. Temporary insanity. Unless you were recently shipwrecked on a deserted island, this should never be you.

1. Hungry. "Hmm . . . I want to eat." Good, real, hearty appetite. Drop in blood sugar levels may make you a touch irritable and mildly lethargic. Possible stomach growling. Go on and eat something yummy.

2. Peckish. "I could nibble on something but it had better be worth it." Slightly hungry—you have a twinge to eat something, but could quite easily hold out longer, too. Eat if it's really worth it—beluga caviar, lobster, white truffle pasta, fresh bluefin tuna, and wagyu beef? Or if eating later will not be possible. Warning: potential risk of emotional eating.

3. Satisfied. "'Twas good and just enough." This is the point of pleasure, the Naughty ideal—a sexy and comfortable fullness. Eating beyond this point would not be related to real hunger but, rather, boredom, greed, or social and/or emotional factors. Warning: eating more could scupper sexual desire. Get a doggie bag—on the double!

4. More than satisfied. "I ate too much." Ever so uncomfortably full. You didn't quit while you were ahead. Your dress may feel tighter and you could feel slightly sluggish. Warning: stop now to escape a binge.

5. Stuffed. "I never want to eat again!" The opposite extreme of famished. Your distended belly makes you feel "food preggers." If you reach this point, you know you've hit bottom, all the more reason to bounce back up without stressing. Warning: high risk of guilt and regret. Banish it! (Refer back to Chapter 2!)

Naughty Appetite Suppressants

Believe it or not, *hunger and appetite* are not synonyms. In fact, they're entirely different processes. *Hunger* refers to the physical need for food in response to chemical changes in the body. *Appetite*, on the other hand, is just the desire to munch—a knee-jerk response to heated emotions, boredom, or perhaps just being around food that looks or smells tasty. While the former keeps us alive, the latter keeps us, well, fatter. When you want to eat but you're not truly hungry, here's what to do instead:

1. Do the perfect red lip.

2. Get a manicure.
   (What better way to preoccupy your hands?)

3. Have sex. With yourself.
   (Okay, maybe this beats a mani . . .)

4. Call an old friend.
   A chatty one.

5. Sort out your Spotify playlists.

6. Then throw an Awesome dance party for one.
   (Preferably in your knickers. Who wants to binge on chicken wings seminude?)

7. Browse a Julia Child cookbook for a new, classically naughty recipe for dindin.
   (Could be a dessert, I won't tell.)

8. Make said new recipe. Share it with someone special, when you *are* hungry.

9. Take a bubble bath.
   (See page 191 for my luxurious recipe.)

10. Go to the gym. LOL.

Let's Play Cravings Cop

Your hardwired hunger DJ is pretty good at spinning healthy-sexy beats. But on rare occasions, she'll freestyle in a way that doesn't support your Naughty weight-loss goals or adhere to your high food standards. And on those occasions, it pays to play the role of cravings cop. Like when . . .

You're PMS-ing: Magnesium levels dip before your period, which can bring on intense cravings for sweets and carbs. The Naughty news is that dark chocolate is one of the richest sources of the mineral. Pregame the painters and buy a box of the best-quality artisanal dark chocolate truffles your money can afford. Treat yourself to one every day for a week. Who says periods have to suck?

You've had a really crappy day: Serotonin, your "happy" hormone, is low, so you'll crave cookies and ice cream for an instant spike. And then you'll overeat, listen to Adele, and do something stupid like overpluck your eyebrows. Do yourself a favor and hit up happy hour for a glass of rosé and a dozen oysters instead. The wine will relax you and the oysters are proven to boost serotonin and help beat the blues. Plus, stepping out is sure to lift your mood, especially if you get good (looking!) service.

You're drunk: Science suggests that alcohol stimulates the appetite in a way that makes you crave high-fat, salty foods. It's no wonder bar snacks are typically a selection of salted nuts, olives, and chips. If you must eat, popcorn is the naughtiest bet: you'll satisfy your need to mindlessly munch on a lot of something salty and buttery for a fraction of the cals and fat grams as a bowl of salted peanuts. Plus the complex carbs will help you sleep/pass out nicely.

Step 6

FIND YOUR
P-SPOT

OLD RULE:
Nothing beats an orgasm.

NAUGHTY WAY:
No foodgasm, no orgasm.

NE NIGHT, at the end of a long dinner in downtown Manhattan with a handful of close friends, I broke a cardinal social rule.

I was seated next to a billionaire investor—a tall, handsome media entrepreneur who was also the fittest fifty-year-old you will ever meet. He had been dazzling the table with stories of his time in L.A. as a movie studio executive, and about the charity work he was doing and the young business people he was mentoring. By his side was his beautiful philanthropist wife who was sharing photos of their children. He was inspiring–here was a man who had a wonderful family, a deeply ingrained value system, a real love of helping others, and a unique perspective on the world that he was willing to share with us.

But there was something I couldn't resist asking him. Letting the red wine flow, I actually turned to this elegant and refined man and spoke the question that everyone wants to ask a self-made billionaire, but is afraid to:

"What's the secret to getting super wealthy?"

I'll never forget the way he smiled at me, and the gracious way he handled that blunt question. Then he leaned in close and shared the simplest strategy I'd ever heard:

"Research everything. Fail and bail. And when you've got a winner, double down."

Fail and bail. And when you've got a winner, double down. It seems so simple! My friend had started dozens of companies, often many at once, investing and divesting quickly and gathering the knowledge he needed to spot the winners. And he had made tens of millions of dollars, not just once, but over and over again.

Yet look at how many of us fail and don't bail–we keep following the same losing strategies, blaming ourselves, and swearing that next time, we'll be smart enough, strong enough, "good" enough. We think the problem is us.

But it's not.

The more I posted about my new approach to food, the more my social media channels blazed hotter than Leo DiCaprio floating on a bed of chocolate. (With me on top.)

We were all setting ourselves up for Food Guilt. And Guilt was making us unhealthy. I resolved that I'd do the research; that I'd bail on what kept failing (no matter how many diet gurus told us we had to be "good"); and that I'd double down when I found the winner.

And how you can win–what I recognized intuitively on that summer's day in St. Tropez, what each of us already knows deep in our heart–is by finding your P-Spot.

P–SPOT, Also termed Pleasure, the P–Spot is vital to a nutritionally complete dining experience and a sexy, flexi body. Turned on by both edible and nonedible sources, the P–Spot can be teased out using the series of protocols in **the Naughty Diet**. Most women don't know where theirs is, or once knew and have since been brainwashed to forget, causing symptoms including but not limited to feeling fat and miserable.

Why is the P-Spot so important? You see, the nutritional advice you get in most diet books ends shortly after the list of forbidden foods and steamed greens meal plan, and somewhere before the calorie calculators come out. And they're all bloody useless. Because what the authors–the "diet experts"– lack is a basic understanding of our basal desire to feel good. Really good.

And most of us don't know how to do it, either. I know because I asked.

"Ladies," I queried in the Naughty Survey, "pick the one overriding, dominating factor when choosing what to eat throughout the course of your week."

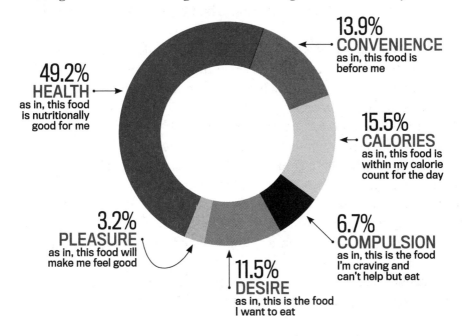

13.9%
CONVENIENCE
as in, this food is
before me

49.2%
HEALTH
as in, this food
is nutritionally
good for me

15.5%
CALORIES
as in, this food is
within my calorie
count for the day

3.2%
PLEASURE
as in, this food will
make me feel good

6.7%
COMPULSION
as in, this is the food
I'm craving and
can't help but eat

11.5%
DESIRE
as in, this is the food
I want to eat

Naughty Activity
SWEAR YOUR HEAD OFF

Turn up the music and shout profanities at failed diet attempts.

PLEASURE, BROADLY SPEAKING, refers to the mental state of feeling good. But it's more than a toe-curling happy ending. Pleasure is a biological imperative. Every living organism, be it the frisky lover in your bed or the finicky orchid on your bedside table, is wired on a cellular level to seek out Pleasure and avoid Pain. It's natural selection at its naughtiest. (That Darwin was such a Naughty one . . .)

When we eat, we are seeking Pleasure from food to avoid the pain of feeling hunger. In other words, Pleasure is key to balancing our appetite. Pleasure, in fact, can help you lose weight.

If this sounds like hedonistic hokum, it's not. I did the research, as my friend advised. (You don't get advice from a billionaire and ignore it.) Here's what the science says:

The P-Spot makes food more nutritious. In a famous study from the 1970s, reported in the *New York Times*, two groups of women—one Swedish and the other Thai—were fed spicy Thai food. The Thai group absorbed more iron—nearly 50 percent more!—than the Swedes.[1] The authors conclude it's because they liked it more. "The Swedish women liked the meal but considered it very spicy," they wrote. "It might be that the strong spices in some way interfered." When both groups were fed the same meal, but all mushed up, the Thai ladies absorbed 70 percent less than the first time. And when they were both fed burgers and mashed potatoes, like the kind you might find at IKEA, the Swedes absorbed more. "The consistency and/or appearance of the food for some reason is of importance for the absorption of iron from the meal," wrote the authors.

What does that teach us? First, if you ever get asked out by a tall blond named Lars, do not suggest Thai food. But also, as the authors concluded, the less you enjoy your food, the less nutritious it is. Your bland, boring "diet" food may be more nutritionally correct when it's on the plate, but what happens inside your body is another thing entirely. Pleasure makes meals more nutritious; remove it, and the nutritional value of food plummets.

The P-Spot makes us happy. According to *Slate*, "One experiment, done with mice genetically altered to be unable to taste sugar, found they still preferred sugar water over plain. Somehow their guts were signaling their brains, sending a 'this is good!' message through some neural backchannel. The mice could not savor the sweetness, yet somehow they were drawn to it just the same!"[2]

The P-Spot makes us leaner. Naughty Girl Marie Antoinette, rumored to regularly let *herself* eat cake for breakfast, would like this bit of research from the Naughty files: dieters who ate dessert for breakfast lost 15 pounds over the course of a sixteen-week program, while participants who ate a small "healthy" breakfast *gained* an average of 24 pounds.[3] So, eat dessert for breakfast? No, that's not the point. The researchers who conducted the study reported that the reason the dessert eaters were able to lose weight was simply that they had given themselves permission to enjoy pleasure foods otherwise "forbidden" by traditional weight-loss plans.

The P-Spot makes life worth living. A Cornell Food and Brand Lab study, published in the journal *Obesity*, asked 501 women about what they eat. Those who were more adventurous and ate out-there ingredients, like seitan or beef tongue, had lower BMIs and felt more passionately about cooking.[4] "There's a real advantage to liking and trying a lot more food," said the study's coauthor, Brian Wansink. "It might even mean you have a lot more fun in life!"

Way to go, you might think at first glance: Half of us want to be healthy! But look how many eat for pleasure. It's one thing to be virtuous; another thing to be a septa from *Game of Thrones*.

Finding pleasure in every bite is what allows perfectly proportioned Naughty girls to indulge in rich desserts, glorious carbs and lethal cocktails without the compulsion to overeat, undereat, purge, run a marathon, run away, hide away, call a therapist, abuse alcohol, swear off alcohol, swear off sugar, swear off men . . . or just swear generally.

We are born Pleasure-seekers.
It's not just the calories that fill us up,
but the Pleasure we get from eating them.
#NaughtyTweet

Find Your P-Spot

WHEN I TELL WOMEN that the key to losing weight and staying healthy is to experience more Pleasure, I often get pushback.

Many women–I'd go so far as to suggest most women–fear their P-Spots. Especially when it comes to food. That's understandable. Submitting to Pleasure means letting go of the thing you want most of all: control. Letting go of the rules and restrictions that traditional diets insist are the be-all and end-all of weight loss makes us afraid that we're walking right into the eye of a massive food binge, one that will cause our thighs, and our self-esteem, to explode. Eating for Pleasure is a truly frightening concept!

But it needn't be. A low Pleasure tolerance makes it hard to get out of our head and to savor our senses. And even though the Naughty approach to eating requires full submission to Pleasure, it does not mean losing control. Nor does it mean you can subsist on Oreos and Red Bull and walk around looking like Gisele. Eating for Pleasure–by definition–means eating for Quality. And when we eat for Quality, we can't help but eat for Health, too.

Not all of us can afford white-truffle honey with every breakfast and chateaubriand at every dinner. But pleasure and quality don't just mean expensive foods in exotic locations. They mean truly embracing and enjoying your food experience.

One expert on pleasure (and quality) I respect is Amber Madison, MA, a noted therapist, author, and lecturer on sexuality, and the relationships columnist for *Men's Fitness.* When I told Amber about Team Naughty, she saddled up quickly. As a leading proponent on the power of pleasure, she has some serious thoughts about its role in our lives.

"In our society, especially in the US, there's this idea that pleasure comes with a price," Amber told me. "Consider sex. Here are the messages we hear when we're teenagers: if you have sex you're gonna get an STD, you're gonna be a slut, you're gonna get pregnant. There's never any discussion as to the good things that may come from pleasure. Sex = pleasure = more sex = bad. It's not till women get older that they start to realize these messages are total bullshit, but the problem is by then you're stuck in your ideas. Pleasure has become somehow dangerous and something we should fear. If you look at the countries where they do female circumcision, that's all about taking pleasure away from women." And while that's the extreme, it's about society (read: men) controlling women; they're afraid that when women control their own pleasure, they control their own life.

"I think too, with food, there's this idea of no pain, no gain," Amber continued. "That being on a diet means you're miserable, and if you're not miserable, then you're not eating healthy. It couldn't be further from the truth.

"I believe if you're having a physical craving, you should give in to it; but some cravings for food aren't physical, they're emotional," she says. "For instance, I used to get intense cravings for sweets after something upsetting or frustrating happened. I know that now, and I can monitor it. If I'm ever really craving something sweet, I double-check myself. If I have a strong craving for something that feels unhealthy I'll do an emotional scan: Am I tired? Am I upset? Am I procrastinating or bored? If I can say no to all those things, I'll indulge my craving. Sometimes a packet of M&Ms really is just the thing. But if I realize I'm actually upset, or otherwise emotionally preoccupied, I'll remind myself that the M&Ms aren't going to make me feel any better, and I probably won't enjoy them either because I'm not in a relaxed state. My body is not fully able to experience pleasure."

Listening to Amber, I started to think that if women want to take control of their weight and their eating habits, they should stop consulting diet gurus and start listening to sex therapists! In fact, the same thing you might say about sex, you can say about food. "Eating right" is sort of like having monogamous missionary-position sex every other Wednesday at 10 p.m. But a woman's needs are more complex than that.

"People like to put things in boxes," Amber says. "*A one-night stand is bad.* Well, what if you're somewhere really romantic and you know a relationship is not feasible but you have an amazing 24 hours connecting with someone and you sleep with them. That's never something to feel bad or guilty about. It was a rich and nourishing experience."

That was it: I wanted my body to be able to experience pleasure from eating, the same way it experienced pleasure from sex! Sometimes I wanted slow and luxurious, and sometimes I wanted a down-and-dirty quickie. And in both sex and food, either approach was okay–as long as it was what I truly wanted. What I chose. And enjoyed guilt-free. Another very Naughty woman I respect had the same thought:

"There is a lustiness that comes with eating passionately, and it's kind of an indicator that you do other things passionately as well," says Cheryl Kramer Kaye, executive beauty director at *Shape* magazine, whose column, "Cheryl Overshares," may be the naughtiest take on beauty you'll ever read. "What it all comes down to with men is sex. Everything that they're seeing translates to, what does this mean in the bedroom? If you can literally let your hair down, or put it up to get it out of the way, that says something about who you are in bed. You can truly enjoy yourself. You have passion. Spontaneity. Who wants to be with the woman who can't accept pleasure from food? No foodgasm, no orgasm.

"I have a dermatologist friend who swears the best thing you can do for your skin is have an orgasm," says Cheryl. "The muscles in your face relax, you get increased blood flow to your cheeks, you get a huge rush of happy feel-good hormones. An orgasm is the ultimate pleasure, and there's a reason women look so great when they get out of bed. A little tousled and flushed . . . "

Okay, okay, I'm sold! I decided to make Pleasure my diet MO, and Quality my guiding light.

It's All About SOUL

I RID MY FRIDGE AND PANTRY of anything my grandmother wouldn't be able to identify, and filled my kitchen with SOUL food–that is, Seasonal, Organic, Unrefined, Local produce. Real food. If it didn't spoil within a week, I never bought it again. I sought out a local farmers' market, made friends with the butcher and fishmonger at my neighborhood grocers (they always gave me the best cuts for the best deals), and spent my weekends tracking down the most delicious fresh bread and local cheeses the city's talented artisans had to offer. Bread and cheese was my kind of fast food.

When I started eating for Quality, food became infinitely more pleasurable–and maintaining my best figure had never been easier. I stopped counting calories, simply because the fresh foods I was buying didn't have labels. My cravings for chocolate dissipated because I actually savored a bite of the real damn thing after lunch instead of wolfing down a packet of no-fat "chocolaty" diet clusters *for* lunch. I started to crave healthy foods. French fries had nothing on the seasonal beets with creamy Gorgonzola salad at my favorite café. And while I still enjoyed the occasional frites and dessert, I got more Pleasure from smaller portions.

I started to think about my diet like my wardrobe. Where bingeing on gallons of Skinny Cow and bags of Skinny Pop became the equivalent of buying the entire sale rack at Forever 21; splurging on a soupcon of foie gras and a glass of champagne at a corner bistro was like leaving Bergdorf with a Dolce LBD. The former would leave me feeling and looking cheap and crappy, whereas the latter made me feel and look like a million bucks. You see, food is like any luxury: The more high-end and luxurious the product, the more valuable it is. And while I understand not everyone can afford an Hermès coat, *everyone* can afford to invest in a perfectly ripe avocado.

Still, I couldn't go without the occasional junk food indulgence–and I do mean junk food. And I realized that stuff like M&Ms and frozen pizzas could fit into my philosophy of Naughty–but only if I truly wanted them. To keep Food Guilt completely out of my kitchen, I needed to check my internal cupboard. How do we know when we're eating for pleasure, and when we're eating for other reasons (reasons that sometimes are closer to self-punishment)? Here are the three-step Pleasure Principles that can guide your decision-making process, and separate indulging (good) from guilt (bad).

Pleasure Principle #1: Tease out universal "facts" from learned beliefs. We have these ideas like "cake is bad," that we think are objective truths in the world. The reality is, these beliefs that we have–about cake, about alcohol, about sex–are learned messages we've heard growing up. It's important to start separating out what's a universal fact, and what's a belief. That can help to soften the rigid borders that can block pleasure, especially when it comes to diet where so few, if any, "rules" will pass the always-true-across-the-board test.

Pleasure Principle #2: Think about the messages you were told about food and eating while growing up. Was your mother always saying, "Oh my god, I can't eat that; it will make me fat"? Perhaps these ideas aren't even yours, but what you saw or heard while growing up. So much of our relationship with food is nurture based; it's learned–culturally and from our family, and then from the media, too. But your food choices are yours, and you don't have to mindlessly repeat patterns you've learned by osmosis. You can relearn and reteach yourself beliefs about food that are helpful and nourishing. You are in control.

Pleasure Principle #3: Understand that letting go does not mean losing control. You can spend your entire life trying to control your diet and maintain the "perfect" body by living a "clean" and "virtuous" food life. When you die, you're not going to get a medal. And you've probably missed out on a ton of Pleasurable experiences, not to mention foodgasms. Life is meant to be enjoyed, and you only get one life! Men are attracted to women who are free with themselves and allow themselves to indulge and feel Pleasure!

When I jumped into the Naughty research as to why the real-deal Quality foods were so integral to Pleasure, why I and so many others who follow the Naughty

Steps have no trouble maintaining our weight no matter what we eat, and why mass-produced diet "food" was so *franken* scary, I was even more convinced that Pleasure and Quality worked hand-in-hand to help us slim down:

- **TRUTH:** A calorie is not a calorie. A study by Harvard researchers that looked at over 120,000 healthy women and men over the course of twenty years found that weight gain was most strongly associated with heavily processed foods as compared to "high-quality" foods of the same caloric value.[5] A hundred calories of Laughing Cow does not equal 100 calories of Camembert. No joke.

- **TRUTH:** Real-deal desserts are more pleasurable. A 50:50 ratio of fat to sugar yields the greatest endorphin release in the body—the real-deal foodgasm, according to a study in *Physiology & Behavior*.[6] Tell me again how much you LOVE that no-fat, sugar-free chocolate pudding? Sorry, I didn't hear you, I was carbogasming over this soufflé.

- **TRUTH:** Artificially sweetened foods hinder our body's natural ability to estimate calorie intake, making it more likely for us to overeat. Rats fed food with artificial sweetener ate three times(!) as much as rats fed regular chow sans creepy sweetener.[7] Skinny Cow? More like Chubby Cow.

- **TRUTH:** Calorie-free sweeteners are creepy. A study in the journal *Diabetes Pro* found that people who drank two or more artificially sweetened diet sodas a day had waist size increases that were six times greater than those of nondrinkers.[8] Yes, your Diet Coke fetish is worth at least two dress sizes.

- **TRUTH:** Calorie-laden sweeteners may be creepier. Princeton University researchers found rats fed high-fructose corn syrup (a cheap sweetener you'll find in most store-bought sweets and even pasta sauces) gained 48 percent more weight than those fed the caloric equivalent of table sugar.[9] And let's face it, store-bought sweets are at least 48 percent less tasty than the real thing. Double the damage, half the fun.

- **TRUTH:** Paying top dollar for naturally slimming foods pays you back. Thin women make a whopping $22,283 more per year than their overweight peers, according to researchers at the University of Florida.[10] For American women, gaining 25 pounds results in an average salary differential of $15,572. (That's two cashmere Hermès coats or one Birkin—Naughty math!)

Healthy food is inherently pleasurable–and if it's not pleasurable, it's not healthy (even if it has the word *diet* on the label). A food that's in season, locally sourced, prepared with love, and beautifully presented on a plate is pleasurable. But "blissful truffle ice cream" that calls itself skinny? You've shortchanged your metabolism and settled. You've faked a foodgasm! Okay, yes. Junk food, even some diet foods, can bring us an occasional jolt of pleasure, but real foods bring even more. And lasts much, much longer.

This was getting exciting. Even as I wrestled my own Food Guilt demons to the ground and pinned them with a Manolo, I was seeing how other women were starting to rally to the cause. I decided I'd devise a fully stocked cupboard and fridge so we could all eat with Pleasure. Check out the next chapter for your Very Naughty Kitchen!

THE LUST SUPPER

11 Naughty (but Guilt-Free) Ways to Push the Pleasure Needle into the Red

The more pleasure you get from your food, the more nutrition you get as well. But pleasure doesn't come just from the food itself, but from the way in which we eat it–the places and people who surround us as we sup. From the Naughty research files, here are 11 ways to relax into the Pleasure hot zone–for zero calories (not that we're counting!)

DON YOUR SEXIEST CHEF'S WHITES. Playing Betty Crocker may enhance the pleasure you get from the finished product. A study published in the journal *Psychological Science* found people who prepared themselves a glass of lemonade reported the drink far tastier than did those who watched someone else whisk together the same recipe.[11]

ADOPT A FEASTING RITUAL. There's no wrong way to eat a bar of chocolate– as long as you have a way that's yours. Feasting rituals, research suggests, are a form of "mindful eating," which has the power to make food more satisfying, and may help prevent overeating. Break off a piece, then close your eyes and savor the flavor. You deserve this!

MAKE EVERY DAY YOUR BIRTHDAY. What's worse for your waistline than a big slice of cake? A big slice of cake with a side of Food Guilt! A study in the journal *Appetite* found people with a weight-loss goal who associated chocolate cake with feeling guilty were less successful at losing weight compared to those who associated the indulgence with celebration.[12] So, stick a candle in it, Naughty Girl, even if it's not your birthday.

STOP TO SMELL THE ROSÉ. The smell of a fine wine or rich dessert can make your mouth water–and may help you eat less, too. A study in the journal *Flavour* found participants ate significantly less of a dessert that smelled strongly of vanilla than they did a mildly scented variety. Researchers say delicious food smells signal to the brain that food is richer, higher in calories, and, consequently, more filling.[13]

SIT DOWN BEFORE YOU CHOW DOWN. Eating while standing up triples caloric intake while simultaneously depleting pleasure from every meal, according to a study conducted numerous times in my own kitchen . . . often after a few too many glasses of wine. Learn from my mistake! Sit down before you eat, even if it's just a quick snack of baby carrots and hummus. And when you're dining out, eat near a window. People who sat near the front of the house "on display" ate the healthiest, according to research by Cornell's Food & Brand lab director Brian Wansink in his book *Slim by Design*.[14]

SET THE MOOD. Cool jazz, low lights–yes, it's time to get romantic, even if you're eating a piece of toast by yourself for brekkie. A study in the journal *Psychological Reports* found that customers who dined in a relaxed environment with dimmed lights and mellow music ate 175 fewer calories per meal (again, not that we're counting) than if they were in a more typical chain restaurant environment.[15] Pull out the candelabra and put on some Barry White, You Sexy Thing!

USE YOUR IMAGINATION. Before grabbing a handful of M&M's, think about what you're about to do. A recent study suggests fantasizing about eating an entire packet of your favorite candies before you indulge may cause you to eat fewer of them.[16] Incredibly, those who imagined eating the most M&M's actually ate the least. Researchers say the findings show that part of the satisfaction we get from food comes from our imagination. So, flex your mental muscles and let that chocolate melt in your mind—not in your mouth.

How to Love the Wine You're With

I use *all my senses* when drinking wine.

I *look* at the label, complete with the vintage, name, appellation, and other details.

I *touch* the bottle to check the temperature is to my liking.

I *hear* the wine open as the cork pops out. Mmm . . . music to my ears.

I *see* the wine, as I pour a drop in the glass. I *hold* the glass at a perpendicular angle to observe the color and texture—this tells me a lot about the age, balance, and body of the wine.

To *smell* the wine, I give the glass a swirl. This releases the bouquet. I nose it once, maybe twice or even thrice, depending on the complexity of notes.

After a good sniffy sniff . . .

. . . I finally *taste* the wine, letting it linger at the front and back of my palate as I "chew" it before swallowing. I experience all the flavors, the length of the notes as well as the texture of the tannins and the finish, be it long or short, complex or not. All being well (no corkage), everyone's glass is filled . . .

I *hear* the high-octave clinks as we raise our glasses in cheers!

I drink merrily but not so hastily that I don't taste the changes in my breathing, living glass of red wine—each sip more open and seductive than the last.

PLATE IT PRETTY. Taking time to make a plate of food look delicious is all part of the enjoyment, researchers say. One study found that a "balanced and artistic" presentation of food was perceived as far tastier than the same meal that looked like something the cat brought up.[17]

GET YOUR PLEASURE'S WORTH. When eating out, you will not be helping to fight World Hunger by cleaning your plate and the chef will not be insulted if you don't finish every morsel. And yeah, I know eating out is not cheap. But neither is diabetes. It's more important to get your pleasure's worth (or a doggy bag) than your "money's worth." Remember, you're paying for the full culinary experience, so it's not a waste just to taste.

THE PIG IS NOT INVITED. Nothing ruins a special dinner out more than the PIG–that's post-indulgence-guilt. On a date, the PIG is a turnoff. Out with the girls, the PIG is a buzz-kill. So, leave the PIG at home. It's rude not to.

PICK YOUR FAVORITE. I often order two appetizers in place of an entrée, especially if I'm saving space for dessert. That's because I'd rather taste a little of a lot. On the whole, restaurant appetizers tend to be more interesting and mouthwatering. Never be shy to order what you really, really want. A glass of red wine, even if everyone else is drinking white wine or not drinking–sure, why not! The Naughty Girl gets what she wants and leaves the dinner table fully satisfied.

EAT NAUGHTY FOODS

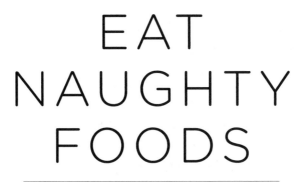

OLD RULE:
Choose diet food that supports your weight loss.

NAUGHTY WAY:
Choose quality food that supports your desires.

THE MOST FREQUENTLY asked question I receive via the Naughty Diet is, *What exactly should I eat?*

And my answer is, you tell me.

Now, wait. Do not throw the book at the wall and pout.

Okay, if you already threw the book, go and pick it up. I'll wait here.

I know what you're thinking: I've teased and seduced you six chapters deep into this tome, and now I'm sending you on with the dietary equivalent of blue balls. But it's not like that, I swear. In this chapter, I'm not going to tell you exactly what to eat. But I am going to help you to figure out on your own exactly what your body wants you to eat—and I'll be right here to guide you to the foods that matter.

What most diet books do is segregate food into categories that are either "superfoods" or "forbidden foods." You eat exactly this number of superfoods, exactly this many times a day, and you avoid the forbidden foods like the plague.

But those protocols are impossible. First of all, I don't have any faith in so-called superfoods. If a food is going to tout itself as a superfood, it better come with a costume. I want to see a stalk of broccoli wearing a kale cape and little tights made from flax meal. And maybe a codpiece. And second of all, I don't believe in forbidden foods–surely you must know that about me by now.

What I believe in is forming a deeper relationship with food, with pleasure, and with the genius in your own body. Only you know which foods and portions support your desires. And it's only by listening to yourself–not to me–that you will come to learn exactly what those foods are, and how much your body wants you to eat of them.

In fact, when it comes down to exactly what to eat, let this be your mantra:

Eat Naughty food.

Limit Nasty food.

And avoid anything Neurotic.

Let me explain what I mean by *Naughty, Nasty, and Neurotic.*

What Makes a Food "Naughty"?

QUALITY.

Quality foods are SOUL foods. That is to say they're seasonal, organic, unrefined, and local. And yet we often shortchange ourselves on meals, slurping up a dinner of ramen to save for that dress. Invest in your body, not what you wrap it in: choosing foods that influence every cell in your body is no time to settle.

That's because quality has real slim-down power. When food lacks the nutrients that we require, the brain senses these shortcomings and responds primitively: *Need more nutrients. Eat more food.*

When you choose cheap, nasty food that's packed with fillers, additives, and what journalist Michael Pollan calls "food-like substances," you confuse your body; it goes into panic mode and tries to store fat. In fact, new research suggests that artificial additives in our food may hinder our body's natural ability to estimate calorie intake, making it more likely for us to overeat.

It's easy to wave the white flag and lament that "everything's killing me, so eff it, pass the Fritos!" or to slide down Neurotic Canyon and control and scrutinize every calorie for fear of premature death (more on this to come). But neither giving up nor clenching up are the best path forward. The Naughty takeaway is this:

Letting quality be your guide gives you the best chance that the food will be Naughty and healthy, whether you're eating carrots, cupcakes, or caviar. Eat for Quality, and you can't help but eat for Pleasure and Health.

Naughty Food Is Freshy Fresh

I KNOW IT SOUNDS like common sense, to focus on what's fresh if you're trying to be healthy. But spare me the eye rolls. I once bought a bag of "fresh" bagels from the supermarket, tossed it on a high shelf in the pantry by accident, and found them ten months later—good as new. Not a speck of mold. They were still soft! I was horrified. Naughty foods aren't just fresh because that's what the store manager decided to put on display today. They are fresh in the freshest sense. They're so fresh they have to live with their auntie and uncle in Bel Air.

To be blunt: Naughty Food rots. Today's baguette should be tomorrow's lethal weapon—hard as a mallet. If a bagel can survive, unscathed, for nearly a year on a high shelf in a Manhattan apartment, just imagine what havoc it can wreak on your poor body while you're trying to digest it. Remnants may still be sitting in our stomach when we die! They may even survive cremation! The key to weight loss is eating Naughty Foods that instantly and effortlessly flood the system with slow-burning nutrition and quick-fire pleasure. These are fresh foods.

There's another reason fresh foods are naughty. When you eat only what's fresh, you are forced to be flexible and sensible. That is to say, you're making food choices with your senses, based on what looks, smells, and feels ripe, ready, and flourishing; not just what some forced algorithm of superfoods in the diet book says you should be eating.

The Naughty Girl isn't going to settle for pale, bland beefsteak tomatoes in February, or rock-hard pears that have spent a week on a ship from Chile. She will make friends with the butcher and the cheese guy at her local grocery store if it means she'll get a slightly choicier cut. She'll happily spend a weekend morning at the farmers' market, rummaging through bins of organic vegetables, smelling the apples, inspecting a cantaloupe, and eating an olive with her full attention. In the end, she won't make ratatouille as planned, because the eggplant and zucchini were looking tired.

There is something spontaneous about eating what's fresh that sings to the Naughty Girl's spirit. She plans for this improvisation and improvises with her plan.

Naughty Tip

**Invest in a big, beautiful basket to
tote home all your goodies.
You'll feel *très* elegant walking home
with a fresh baguette and a bunch
of kale peeking out from the top,
and less inclined to choose foods that fail
the fresh test. There is nothing chic
about a basket heaving with
frozen pizza boxes . . . however nice
the basket.**

Naughty Foods Don't Have Calories

Screw the calories and pass the wine. #NaughtyTweet

IMAGINE IF WE VIEWED our friends the way so many of us view our food: as a list of numbers. Supposing I stopped calling you by your first name and started calling you 150 (your weight), or 1,700 (calories consumed yesterday) or 2,600 (square footage of your home). You would hate it! And you'd hate it, because you would assume I had reduced you to an arbitrary figure that tells me nothing about what kind of a person you are, a number that in the end is inconsequential to our friendship. There are plenty of people who do flash these sort of figures around and choose social circles based upon them (plus net worth, number of homes, diamond karats, ccs of collagen . . .). Naughty girls aren't those kind of people, and don't enjoy schmoozing with them, either.

When you choose foods based on their calorie content alone, you further distance yourself from the genius in your body and its ability to tell you exactly what it needs to look and feel its very best. Your body doesn't speak "calorie." When's the last time you had a craving for "100 calories of almonds, please!"? Your body speaks the language of pleasure. Choose the quality foods that turn you on, and your body will take care of the rest.

But, M! If I ate nothing but the highest-quality hand-dipped chocolate almonds all day I wouldn't fit through my front door! you say.

Of course, we need to be aware of the energy density of foods. But as we already discovered in chapter 5, the brain in your belly has the profound ability to practice perfect portion control for you. It is almost impossible to overeat on raw fruits and vegetables; and equally challenging to eat piles of chocolate-covered almonds all day long. But Cheetos, White Castle sliders, Doritos, Sonic slushies, or one of those monster mix-ins from Cold Stone? That's hard-core junk, and you can see the bottom of the cup, bowl, or bag faster than you'd ever imagine.

Some Naughty Foods are outrageously decadent–like the flourless chocolate torte I had at Jacques Torres yesterday, for instance–while others provide little energy at all. Like my homemade kale chips that are currently in the oven (yum!). High calorie, low calorie, or somewhere in between–it matters not a jot.

When it comes to reaching and maintaining a healthy-sexy body, all that matters is that you're consistently choosing quality foods that push your pleasure needle to the red.

THINGS TO COUNT INSTEAD OF CALORIES

There are tons of things in life worth counting; calories most certainly aren't one of them.

1. **Lucky stars**

2. **Blessings**

3. **Kisses**

4. **Thread count**

5a. **Compliments given**

5b. **Compliments received (make sure a is always greater than b)**

6. **Bottles of wine left**

7. **Days till your next vacation**

8. **Hours till you see your loved ones**

9. **Deep breaths . . .**

10. **And sheep**

Naughty Food Isn't Nasty
or Neurotic

CHOOSING FRESH, QUALITY FOODS that have a good story to tell is your first and fundamental step to filling your kitchen and your body with Naughty Foods that serve you well. But it's just as important to limit the nonnutrients as it is to include the Naughty ones. What are nonnutrients? They fall into two groups: Nasty and Neurotic.

Nasty and Neurotic foods are the antithesis of Naughty. They are lacking in quality in the truest sense, because they tell a story that is twisted and tortured. They're products of our simultaneous addictions to eating and to dieting.

Nasty foods are born of our inability to practice portion control, and our hardwired preferences for sweets, fats, and salts–three tastes that were hard to come by in the good ol' Flintstone days when we sweated more, ate less, and considered honey and fats rare finds worth bingeing on for survival reasons. Nasty Foods are processed and packaged in such a way we are helpless but to overeat them. They're oversalted; oversized or undersized; stripped of filling fiber; and pumped full of calorie-free sweeteners and preservatives that mess up our satiety hormones. Then they're marketed as quick fixes for everything from a bad day to a bumpy backside. They only make us hungrier, fatter, and more miserable.

On the other end of the spectrum, Neurotic foods are born of a violent reaction to what Nasty foods are doing to our body (bumpy backside at the top of the list). They're stripped of anything that sounds mildly pleasurable and boosted with those much-loathed superfoods. ("My juice cleanse has more green algae extract than your juice cleanse!")

I have nothing against spirulina, whey protein, hemp milk, kale cupcakes, fish oil pills, or energy bars made from crickets. If you have a joyous, fulfilling, and mutually beneficial relationship with food, then adding an extra nutritional boost can only help. But as I've said in previous chapters, your body cannot claim its full nutritional due unless you're enjoying your food experience. Plus, food that turns you on, turns on your metabolism.

Naughty girls like shortcuts, so here are the Cliff's Notes:

Nasty Food

- Contains ingredients preceded by verbs like *modified, reduced,* or *extracted.*

- The words *light, lite, lean, skinny, fat-free, low-calorie,* or *diet* appear on the packaging.

- Contains ingredients you can't find for sale, individually, in a supermarket and certainly won't find growing in a field.

- Sold in neat, 100-calorie controlled packets or, conversely, sold in "king," "super" or "jumbo," or "colossal" -size bags.

- Comes with very long expiration dates, many moons away. Never rots.

- "Artificially flavored" or "sweetened" is a dead giveaway of dead foods.

- The list of ingredients is longer than Lohan's list of lovers.

- Most of the ingredients would make high-scoring Scrabble words; however, you won't find *butylated hydroxyanisole* in the dictionary.

- "Microwave only" meals—be afraid, be very afraid.

- Disney characters on the box or free gifts inside. Walk on by . . .

Neurotic Food

- Seemingly "free" of most things: sugar-free, carb-free, gluten-free, dairy-free, sodium-free, fat-free, calorie-free.

- Weirdly green. Think green granola, spirulina brownies, kale gum.

- Claims to replace a pleasure food. "A protein bar so good you'll never eat chocolate again!"

- Vitamin-enriched.

- Weighed, counted; reweighed and recounted by you.

- Contrived from its original state so as to reduce calories. A scooped-out bagel, for instance.

- Blessed by monks in an exotic country.

- Sourced from a mountain or volcanic range.

- Sold in über-trendy, BPA-free packaging.

- So expensive you can't afford to eat a full serving in one sitting.

- Not tasty; kids would likely spit it out.

So, I Eat What Now?

WHATEVER YOU EAT, aim to eat Naughty foods 80 percent of the time, a classic strategy Maria Menounos (*New York Times* bestselling author of *The EveryGirl's Guide to Life*) has used to great effect–she lost 40 pounds! This guarantees you'll be receiving a majority of high-nutrient, high-pleasure foods that your body needs and craves while significantly reducing the toxins and artificial crap that mess with your hunger hormones, metabolism, digestion and overall well-being.

Keri Glassman, RD, the founder of Nutritious Life and author of a number of books on eating well, including the very naughtily titled *Slim, Calm, Sexy Diet*, put it perfectly when we were on the phone discussing the "naughty middle road" of eating. Her perfectly naughty advice? Think about your diet as you do your finances:

"You want to build good nutritional credit by making regular, high-quality payments to your body. When you have good nutrition credit, you can afford to splurge more or skip a quality meal without terrible consequences. Your body trusts that this is a one-off thing and a more standard payment is on the way. It's when you're constantly making giant calorie payments and then restricting for days that your body says 'screw this!' It's okay for the pendulum to swing. This is life! We have dinner dates and holidays, and these food events can make great memories. We just want to avoid living in the extremes. Focus on feeding your body a steady diet of whole foods on a regular basis and make sure that you're eating the best quality foods you can."

A Naughty girl is sexy flexi. She'll happily enjoy a vegan soup for lunch and a paleo salad for dinner; and console a heartbroken friend in the afternoon with a box of Girl Scout cookies. She'll say yes to more wine and dessert while on holiday in France and damage-control with a short juice cleanse back home. She'll have white rice this week and brown rice next time (because no one likes a rice-ist); kale chips today and Kettle Brand tomorrow. The Naughty Diet doesn't pretend that frozen pizzas don't exist or that snacking on ice cubes never happens. We all have our nasty, neurotic tendencies: that's what the 20 percent margin of erring is for. Because it is always erring, and never an error. Expect to mess up; enjoy messing up; move on.

In fact, when I asked Maria Menounos about her secret to losing 40 pounds–and keeping it off–she told me "cheating" was integral to her success:

"I love loaded potato skins, fries, onion rings and pretty much anything on the appetizer menu at T.G.I. Friday's or Chili's! I also love ice cream. When I eat that stuff I just enjoy it. It doesn't make any sense not to. It's all about compensating the following days, when you go off track. I basically 'clean up' by eating more salads, vegetables and drinking lots of water."

To give you a more detailed idea of Nasty, Naughty, and Neurotic food choices, peruse this list. Understand this is not a list of rules about what exactly to eat, but just a list that, considered collectively, should help you settle into the Naughty middle way of eating . . . most of the time.

What's Vile in the Aisle
A Guide to the Top 50 Naughty Foods

{Dairy}

YOGURT

Nasty Light & Fit, fruit-flavored, "fat-free" = sugar-laden

Naughty Fage Total 0% plain Greek yogurt. Add honey or fresh fruit to sweeten and nuts or granola for a crunchy texture.

MILK

Nasty Shelf-stable milk box

Naughty Anything that's not flavored, sweetened or ultrapasteurized; preference for whole milk sold in bottles (dibs on the cream top). Shoutout to Ronnybrook Dairy Farm's milk.

CHEESE

Nasty 2 or 3 wedges of Laughing Cow

Naughty Knob of Brie

EGGS

Nasty Muscle Egg flavored liquid egg whites

Naughty Organic eggs–all the better if you have to flick away a feather.

BUTTER

Nasty Margarine. I Can Believe It's Not Butter

Naughty Unsalted, cow's milk, preferably French produced. *Beurre d'Échiré* is France's best. When you see it, do not resist.

COTTAGE CHEESE

Nasty Friendship 1% Lowfat Cottage Cheese, with carrageenan,
a binding agent often found in toothpaste

Naughty Breakstone's 4% small curd

{Produce}

FRUIT

Nasty 100-calorie-pack fruit snacks

Naughty Anything and everything organic, local, and in season;
whatever looks, smells, and feels fresh. I've squeezed every melon–go to
naughtydiet.com for a full list of what to buy when.

VEGGIES

Nasty All the ranch-flavored dips, filled with MSG,
they put next to the cucumbers

Naughty Anything on my naughtydiet.com list of veggies
that are in season now

GODDESS GREENS, pertaining to any dark, leafy greens that are essential to feeling goddesslike. Limitless amounts of these supergreens are permitted on the Naughty Diet. It's a case of more is more when eating kale, collards, watercress, bok choy, broccoli rabe, endive, chicory, arugula, and mesclun. The Goddess Greens reign supreme; rich in fiber, folic acid, phosphorous, iron, calcium, potassium, magnesium, zinc, vitamins A, C, E, K, and many more phytochemicals and micronutrients.

{Meat and Fish}

FISH

Nasty Fried tilapia

Naughty I like my fish as I like my men:
anything wild that doesn't smell. Pan-seared wild salmon is
a favorite, or anything cooked en papillote.

BURGERS

Nasty Veggie burger with soy cheese, turkey bacon,
and no bun, no fries

Naughty Go big or go home! Burger time is no time to scrimp,
especially on quality and personal taste.
Look for 100% beef (sirloin for me!) patties,
make sure they're cooked just right for you. Only add toppings
that add high-mileage pleasure. So, if you feel *meh*
about cheese, forget it. But if caramelized onions, a sliver of
crispy bacon, slice of gherkin, dollop of chutney or
bite of foie gras rocks your burger experience, bring it!
The best burgers are made-to-order.

BEEF

Nasty Meat in a box

Naughty Grass-fed meat contains higher levels of omega-3 fatty acids,
according to a study published in *Nutrition Journal*,
which have been shown to reduce the risk of heart disease.[1]

PORK

Nasty Spam, the junk in a can, not your mailbox. And pepperoni,
saturated in fat. Sorry, Five Guys.

Naughty Thinly sliced prosciutto with melon

BACON

Nasty Turkey bacon. Why bother?

Naughty Crispy porkalicious bacon

CHICKEN

Nasty Chicken patties and nuggets–they're often held together
with soy protein, cornstarch, "flavor," MSG, and sugar.
Cluck that shit.

Naughty Organic isn't always worth it,
but in the poultry section, it is.
A recent study comparing conventional, antibiotic-free,
and USDA organic chicken found that inorganic
arsenic concentrations were four times
higher in conventional chicken meat than
in USDA organic chicken.[2]

TURKEY

Nasty Any brand with nitrates, unnecessary preservatives

Naughty White meat fresh off the bone,
with a spot of fatty dark thrown in for flavor.
Or if you're buying packaged slices, go with Applegate Farms.

{Cereals}

OATMEAL

Nasty Quaker weight-control peaches & cream

Naughty Well-made or overnight oats with chia seeds,
Greek yogurt, bananas, walnuts,
and honey (see page 181 for my recipe)

CEREAL

Nasty Anything with the word *chocolaty* or *froot* or *clusters*

Naughty Anything with four or fewer ingredients;
add a drizzle of honey and some berries. Swiss müesli with
no added sugar is tops.

{Snacks}

CANDY

Nasty Skittles. Each colored bead is essentially sugar
and corn syrup glued together with hydrogenated palm kernel oil,
and no less than 10 artificial colors!

Naughty Chupa Chups. And M&M's, well hidden in the fridge.

CHOCOLATE

Nasty Skinny Cow clusters

Naughty One or two of anything bite-size from
a chocolate shop–dark, milk or white; or one Baci or real kiss!

COOKIES

Nasty 100-calorie pack of Oreos

Naughty Home-baked chocolate chip, still warm
from the oven–even Toll House are better than Chips Ahoy

PROTEIN BAR

Nasty Think Thin bars, think not.

Naughty Epic Habanero Cherry Beef Bar.
Sweet, salty, and unexpected.

GRANOLA BAR

Nasty Nutri-Grain strawberry yogurt

Naughty Anything KIND

CRACKERS

Nasty Reduced-fat Wheat Thins

Naughty Carr's crackers. The calories are negligible
and they're a great palate cleanser–plus good
for wine tastings!

CHIPS

Nasty Anything that changes the color of your fingers.
And processed "beige" carbs like bagel chips,
pretzels, and cookies should stay out of eyesight,
in nonclear containers, in another country.

Naughty Popchips or simple potato chips as a side to a healthy meal

---

POPCORN

Nasty Pop Secret–the secret is, *shh,*
it has 5 grams of trans fats!

Naughty Pour a tablespoon of olive oil
into a deep pot, and add a pinch of salt and 1 cup of
loose popcorn kernels. Cover. Shake the pot every few seconds.
Remove from the heat when the pops slow down,
about 4 minutes later. Pair with HBO.

TORTILLA CHIPS

Nasty Any brand that ends with *itos*

Naughty All Garden of Eatin' flavors, especially Chili & Lime.
Give in to temptation.

SQUIRREL FOOD, pertaining to any nuts, seeds, and dried fruit I tuck in my cheeks when cravings strike. Nuts pack a punch of energy and health-hearty fats. They're my go-to snack, especially when I don't have time to eat properly. (An aside: Many weight conscious women fear nuts because they're high in fat calories. But remember our body needs these fats to function optimally. As a kid, I remember a friend telling me that a peanut a day provided enough energy to keep a person alive for weeks on end. Fact or fiction, I fell in love with the power of legumes there and then.)

NUTS

Nasty 100-calorie cocoa almonds

Naughty Walnuts for breakfast;
cocktail peanuts at cocktail hour; pistachios whenever,
because they take a quick minute to remove from their shells

{Condiments}

MAYONNAISE

Nasty Fat-free anything

Naughty Sir Kensington's, especially the Chipotle flavor

MUSTARD

Nasty Bright yellow means caution.

Naughty Grey Poupon, the classic Naughty brand that brought
refinement to the supermarket

SALSA

Nasty Abort Mission

Naughty Newman's, Hot!

SALAD DRESSING

Nasty Anything Walden Farms (calorie-free)

Naughty Balsamic vinaigrette: 3:1 ratio of olive oil to balsamic vinegar.
Season with minced garlic/lemon juice/sea salt/black pepper/
oregano–*amore*!

OIL AND VINEGAR

Nasty Vegetable oil and vinegar, especially if it's white

Naughty Olive oil (extra-virgin preferred), grapeseed oil, canola oil,
sesame oil, and peanut oil (stir-fries will never be the same again!)
As for vinegars, go with balsamic, cider, and red and white wine.
These all add tons of flavor with virtually no calories
(not that we're counting . . .).

SWEETENERS

Nasty The pink stuff. The blue stuff. The yellow stuff.

Naughty Manuka honey, brown sugar, date sugar, molasses, maple syrup,
stevia, agave nectar, and a spoonful of love

{Frozen}

PIZZA

Nasty Tombstone frozen pizza

Naughty Hand-tossed brick-oven margherita with extra fresh basil,
or try my recipe on page 154.

VEGGIE BURGERS

Nasty Morningstar Farms. If you need oil for your Vespa,
microwave one.

Naughty Beyond Meat, the ambitious
new brand of veggie patties,
ground "beef" and "chicken" strips
that's pitching plant-protein products for carnivores.
All the flavor, none of the blood.

PASTA

Nasty Frozen soy mac and cheese bowl

Naughty Half order of spaghetti alle vongole

WAFFLES

Nasty Leggo that Eggo.

Naughty Van's Belgian waffles,
if you can't get to Brussels

ICE CREAM

Nasty Skinny Cow!

Naughty Talenti or any brand of fresh gelato

POPSICLES

Nasty Popsicle

Naughty Whole Fruit Strawberry Bars.
In what has to be a first,
fruit outranks sugar in the ingredients list.
For more pop, turn to page 165
for Naughty Rosé Popsicles.

{Breadstuffs}

BAGELS

Nasty 2 bagel thins with fat-free cream cheese

Naughty Half an everything with lox and
a shmear of cream cheese

BREAD

Nasty Any bread labeled "whole wheat" that lists
"whole wheat" as the second, third, fourth,
or fifth ingredient–after brown sugar.
Pepperidge Farm, I'm talking to you!

Naughty A fresh baguette. Press your thumb into the tip and
if it dents the crust, buy it; if not, run!

PANCAKES

Nasty 4 Special K waffles with
¼ cup Walden Farms calorie-free syrup

Naughty Crepes with fresh lemon juice and
a light dusting of sugar and cinnamon,
or served with fresh cream and berries

PIE

Nasty Mrs. Smith. Get a divorce.

Naughty Petite tartes aux fruits
from a patisserie

CARBOLOAD, To stock one's pantry with healthy, nutrient-dense carbs and grains, like oatmeal, barley, lentils, popcorn (not microwave), beans: black, pinto, kidney, chickpeas, lentils, canned refried beans (for Mexican fiestas) dried peas (green, split, yellow), quinoa, couscous, orzo, ramen noodles, brown rice, and whole wheat pasta–spaghetti and penne are my favorites. All these carbs require cooking, reducing the risk of a spontaneous carb binge. Pita bread and tortilla wraps can go in the freezer–out of sight, out of mouth–and are easily defrosted when needed.

{Ethnic Foods}

SUSHI

Nasty California roll and spider roll, with mayo

Naughty Omakase–chef's choice
(no tempura, please)

PASTA SAUCE

Nasty No Prego

Naughty Newman's Own Marinara Sauce

{Spices}

Nasty The ones you bought when Bush was president, still on the shelf

Naughty A well-stocked spice rack is a Naughty Kitchen essential!
Start filling yours with:

SEA SALT
goes with everything

BLACK PEPPER
blocks fat cells

ROSEMARY
marry it with lamb

BASIL
fresh is always best

OREGANO
not to be smoked

DILL
loves fish

CRUSHED RED PEPPER
flat-out makes you horny

CINNAMON
makes everything taste like a cookie

CHILI POWDER
suppresses appetite

TURMERIC
reduces bloat

CILANTRO
makes your blood pump

CUMIN
try it in yogurt

GARLIC
boosts sex drive (pair with gum)

PAPRIKA
best on devilish eggs

All these herbs and spices have health boosting–and even weight-loss properties and add spice to the Naughty Girl's life!

SUPERSEEDS, Orphans of plants everywhere, superseeds find a better home in my cupboard. Top of the list for Quality is the ch–ch–ch–***chia seed***! It scores high in iron, folate, calcium, and magnesium to promote bone health, heart–healthy omega–3 fatty acids, and cholesterol–lowering soluble fiber that will keep you feeling fuller for longer. I like to add them to smoothies, yogurt, and oatmeal because they turn gelatinous in liquids, making them even more digestible.

{Drinks}

COFFEE[3]

Nasty Venti sugar-free vanilla soy latte with 2 Splenda

Naughty Tall skim vanilla latte, whole milk cappuccino, espresso

TEA

Nasty Diet Snapple iced tea

Naughty Any tea bag that doesn't have artificial flavors (I'm partial to chai, rooibos, peppermint, chamomile, black, green)

WINE[4]

Nasty Anything with calories on the bottle (there is a special circle in hell reserved for these manufacturers.) Anything from a box.

Naughty A big, bold, smooth (soft tannins) cabernet sauvignon– Naughty Girls love big boys! (Rosé in the summer)

JUICE

Nasty "From concentrate"

Naughty Orange juice (expressly for weekend mimosas),
apple juice, and lots of grape juice (fermented and bottled)

MIXERS

Nasty Glow-in-the-dark fruit flavors

Naughty Expired Dayquil and Nyquil for cocktails and colds.
I kid, I kid. Drink mojitos and martinis, and buy accordingly.

WATER

Nasty Vitaminwater

Naughty San Pellegrino or tap water
with sliced citrus fruits

The Naughty Kitchen

SINGLE PEOPLE LIKE to joke about how infrequently they use their kitchen. Especially my single city friends who tend to use their kitchen cupboards–even their fridge–as storage space for Loubs and lotions.

"I don't even know how to turn this thing on," chuckled a male model friend just the other day. "I eat out all the time, you know," he added, while running his fingers across the virgin Wolf stovetop.

Yeah, I do know. My former kitchens were also sad, sorry spaces; filled with lonely crockery, cutlery, and cookware. How many dinner plates did I own? No clue. I lived off the top two. Did I have a paring knife? No clue. I only used one. I moved about my kitchen with the awkwardness of an un-invited guest. It wasn't until I met my dream man, moved to New York, and quite frankly grew up (a little), that I started to use the kitchen as a kitchen.

I want you to start using your kitchen as a Naughty Kitchen. The Naughty Girl knows the power of a good heel and a well-stocked kitchen. Both will make you look and feel hotter. Your kitchen is so much more than just a place of dirty late-night binges (dirty sex, sure) and takeout. Your kitchen is a Zen-den full of sensual pleasures–full of delicious and nutritious tastes, smells, sights, sounds, and textures. Your kitchen is where you can safely satisfy all your cravings, nourish your body, and express yourself through food. Food gives life and cooking it is an expression of love. The Naughty Kitchen is a place to live love and love living.

Here's how to give your kitchen a naughty makeover.

The Naughty Kitchen Must-Haves

Paring knife! Obvi.

Bright and cheerful **fruit bowl** always overflowing with fresh and seasonal, ready washed fruit. Let this be the centerpiece of your kitchen. Let it entice you to have an apple a day before you stray. Stock it with bananas—Nature's energy bar—lemons, apples, oranges, and any other seasonal fruit.

Fresh flowers to stimulate all your other senses, bar taste

Wide selection of **wine and champagne glasses.** The right glass for the right wine.

Blender for superpower smoothies

Juicer, even if unused, it's well intended. Keep it on display to inspire spontaneous juicing.

Spice rack full of spices and herbs that add flavor and health benefits to meals

Reliable **wine opener**

Backup wine opener

Good selection of **plastic bins** so you can quickly and easily store and freeze leftovers.

Water pitcher, filled with inviting lemon- or cucumber-infused ice water—just as you'd find at a swish-swish hotel reception or spa. The Naughty Kitchen is an elegant spot.

Coffee mugs for every mood. I have a full set of *Little Miss* character cups. Suffice it to say; Little Miss Naughty is a regular favorite.

Nonstick pans because they're easy to clean and let you cut back on cooking oil. Home cooking lets you control the oil usage! Restaurants don't give a damn and only want the food to taste good.

Serious **knife set** that screams "I am the Master Chef (and I am dangerous)"

Good **chopping boards** that scream to be abused by your knives

A totally unnecessary **ice pick**, for when basic instinct takes over

Everyday apron for unexpected messes

Clear Out

Throw out all expired/spoiled food, including old frozen food that you know you're never going to eat. This is similar to a wardrobe clearing out. You only want food that you actually want to eat (and should be eating) in your fridge and freezer. Bye-bye, Tater Tots.

Throw out the nastiest takeaway delivery menus. You know, the picture ones covered in greasy finger stains.

Throw out all expired vitamins and supplements, protein powders, green powders, cacao powder. Also toss any big, gelatinous pills that make you barf. (There are other available sources of fish oil.)

Throw out all nasty, highly processed food products. Especially the ones labeled "diet." You know how I feel about those.

Sexy apron for expected messes. ;)

Funny apron because cooking should be fun. Mine says: "All this! And I Can Cook!" on the back.

Oven gloves, to prevent cooking war wounds

Cookbooks, for inspiration and decoration, but improvisation is more the naughty way.

Pretty **place mats** for pretty presentation

Candles to help set the mood and make you look ten years younger

Soda-stream machine, for retro fun and limitless, sparkling concoctions that will fill you up on fat-free fizz. Also, since soda is the devil, better the devil you know.

Steam cooker for the lightest and healthiest way to cook food. Angelina Jolie swears by steam cooking.

Cocktail shaker, for your inner Bond Girl

Egg cups; for soft-boiled eggs with naughty toast soldiers.

Bread bin, because we eat bread!

Bread basket, see above.

Toaster, see above, above.

Toast rack, see above, above, above. The Naughty Kitchen is all about elegance and making food special.

Breakfast tray, for naughty breakfasts in bed

Quality coffee machine. If you're a coffee lover, this is a worth-while investment when you consider a Starbucks costs around $5. To live a charmed and naughty life, drink the finest coffee available. Life is too beautiful and short not to.

Wine decanter. Technically, only old, fine wines need decanting to breathe and release their full bouquet. But I like the ritual of decanting wines—it makes it feel more special. Plus once it's out of the bottle, it's going one place and one place only. Drink one decanter/many bottles. Drink one glass/many pours.

Wine rack to proudly display your art, I mean wine

Wine fridge, to store your wine at the ideal 55°F. A luxury investment.

Oxy Clean, for wine stains, obviously

Things You Won't Find in the Naughty Kitchen

Food Guilt, Fears, and Anxiety

Skinny Cow, Twinkies, and other nasty, highly processed sweets

Shake 'N Bake, Hamburger Helper, and other nasty, highly processed flavorings

Froot Loops, Lucky Charms, and other nasty, milk-color-altering cereals

Nasty, frozen microwave meals

Weight Watchers, Lean Cuisine, and other diet food brands

Special K and other cardboard-tasting foodstuff

Soda, diet or regular

Roaches and rats

Pecan Pie Pringles

Energy bars, protein powders, meal replacement shakes, and energy drinks

Boxed wine

No wine

A fryer

Diet books

A laptop, iPad, or TV. (Music totally allowed and encouraged.)

An empty fridge

Boredom

A salt shaker

Plastic cutlery

Chipped crockery

Vending machine, just saying . . .

Butler, sadly

COOK WHEN YOU WANT

OLD RULE:
1,256, 1,257, 1,258 calories

NEW RULE:
Count on feeling better with every bite.

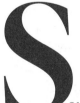

OMEWHERE THERE'S A PLACE that means more to you than anywhere else on earth. It might be the place you are now, the place you grew up, or someplace you visited only once in your life. Think about that place now. Can you see it?

There are people in your life who are sacred to you. Family, friends, lovers, people who inspire and define you. Put those people into that sacred place. Set them around a large table.

There's music playing in the background. Your favorite songs, an evocative mix, large with glorious grooves.

And laid out on that table is a scrumptuous spread.

Hold this moment in your head. We'll come back to it.

Fall Back in Love with Food

FOR MOST OF MY LIFE, I saw food as something that existed in its own realm. It was the ultimate frenemy, taunting and teasing me, promising me joy and then crushing me with feelings of guilt and shame. And because it ate up so much room in my head, it took on a life of its own. I put it "over there," as something to be dealt with, managed, resisted, and feared.

That's the way a lot of us think of food. And that's been our downfall.

We live today in a world where everything needs to be "optimized." The great glut of information at hand allows us to monitor our popularity (ooh, 87 likes!), our success (only $257,000 a year more to hit the 1%!), and our sexual worthiness (did you know women with a hip-to-waist ratio of 0.7 have optimal estrogen levels?). And that means we can calculate the exact ratio of omega-3 to omega-6 in our diet; build meals around "macros" and tweak them for their carb/fat/protein balance; and manage our caloric intake down to the last digit–especially with those handy new placards they've slapped on every chain restaurant menu in America.

And all of this takes food out of our actual, real lives, and puts it "over there," away from our emotional and spiritual lives. We don't define our favorite place by its altitude or its population. We don't choose our loved ones based on their bank account numbers or BMIs (at least, I hope not!). And we don't choose our music by its beats per minute.

Why do we treat our food differently?

Go back to that sacred place. I can't possibly guess the spot you've chosen. It might be the screened-in porch of a fishing cabin in the Louisiana backwater, or a piazza across from a majestic cathedral in Milan, or the gently lapping shores of a Bahamian beach. Only you know. But there's probably food there–shrimp po'boys and beer, or prosciutto and prosecco, or conch ceviche and freshly cut coconut water.

I don't know the people you've invited. But I do know you've undoubtedly shared dozens, maybe thousands of meals with them, and that you've laughed and argued and cried together over meat and bread and drinks.

I can't guess at the music you're playing. But it's a soundtrack that evokes important moments in your life, moments that probably revolved at least in part around food–wild parties or slow, intimate dinners or freewheeling road trips.

So, if I can't tell you the place, the people, or the soundtrack, how can I possibly tell you what food goes on your table?

What I can tell you is what food goes on my table.

My food loves and pleasures me. It makes me look and feel my best. It indulges and satisfies me. It never makes me feel guilty. Our relationship is like the best of romances–it's built on pleasure, passion, spontaneity, compromise, forgiveness, trust, and mutual respect.

The Naughty Menu

I'VE SAID IT BEFORE and I'll reiterate it now: I cannot tell you what to eat. I can't tell you whether you should eat breakfast every day, or skip it altogether. I can't prescribe a set number of calories, or dictate a carb/protein/fat ratio, or profess a miracle plan for lowering your glycemic load.

Or rather, I could do all those things . . . but I'm not going to.

Because it would be hypocrisy to set out a diet plan that I, myself, would never follow. In part, it's because I don't believe in diet plans–diet plans are what got us into the mess to begin with. And in part, it's because my body's needs, and my soul's needs, are simply far different from yours.

The act of eating is an act of communion with one's body. With each bite, you're telling it a story about the food you're consuming–where it came from, why you've chosen it, how it's fitting in with your life. Neither I nor anyone can dictate that tale; it has to come from you.

That said, I can give you a collection of more than 30 of my favorite Naughty recipes–each decadent, healthy, and fun to make.

And at the end of this chapter, I've laid out the Naughty Nutrients; they are the critical ingredients of my daily food intake, and they should be yours as well. And if you want to eat them in three square meals, or in six little round ones, or in one gigantic trapezoid pigfest, that's your prerogative. But here's how I do it:

BREAKFAST

There's a lot to be said for skipping breakfast, especially if you're active in the first half of the day. A 2013 randomized, controlled trial determined that exercising on an empty stomach increased fat burn by 20 percent. On the other hand, eating a combination of fiber, healthy fats, and protein (especially in the form of eggs) seems to help people stay fuller longer, and to actually reduce the number of calories they eat throughout the day.

One thing we do know: An unhealthy breakfast–especially one that's devoid of those three nutrients–is definitely worse for you than skipping the meal altogether. So, dodge Dunkin', circumnavigate Krispy Kreme, and don't get tricked by any sneaky rabbits.

Here are five great breakfasts that are packed with fiber, healthy fats, and protein.

The Green Goddess Smoothie

Serves: 1 / Prep time: 3 minutes / Blend time: 1 minute

ALL YOU'LL NEED:

¼ avocado, peeled and pitted

1 ripe banana

1 tablespoon honey

½ cup brewed green tea

1 scoop protein powder

½ cup ice

1 teaspoon grated fresh ginger (optional)

PUTTING IT TOGETHER:

1. Blend! Fiber and protein combine forces to vanquish any hunger in this untraditional but tasty creation.

The World's Best Scrambled Eggs

This is not a recipe. It's just a guideline to help your breakfast feel decadent and taste incredible. I think that 90 seconds is all that stands between good scrambled eggs and amazing scrambled eggs. Your morning routine can spare 90 seconds and I promise your tummy (and anyone you make breakfast for) will thank you.

1. Use fresh eggs.

This is obvious, but fresh eggs taste better. Egg cartons are marked with a three-digit number–this number is your friend. It corresponds to the date the eggs were packaged, so eggs packaged on January 1 will be coded 001 and eggs packaged on December 31 will read 365. So, check the side of the carton and do the math to get the best eggs possible.

2. Whisk!

Everyone has a favorite way of preparing scrambled eggs, whether that means adding milk or cream or water. . . . If you have a ratio you like, stick with it, but by all means whisk the eggs. I like to use a small whisk and a large bowl and beat the eggs vigorously for a good, Naughty minute.

3. Season.

Add salt and pepper to the eggs before adding them to the pan. It may seem obvious but salt makes a world of difference.

4. Cook the eggs slowly.

This is where the 90 seconds come in. Scrambled eggs are a simple dish and for some reason that seems to imply we should crank up the heat and practically burn them before scarfing them down. The trick is this: just use a much lower heat and swirl the eggs around the pan. That's it!

I usually use a touch of nonstick spray and then pour the eggs into a shallow pan. If I'm making the eggs for myself, I add a pat of butter. The heat should be somewhere between medium and low. You'll know it's right if it takes about 45 seconds before the eggs start to cook. Once the eggs start to set up, use a spatula to move them around the pan, gently move them back and forth. Once they are cooked through–but not dry–your eggs are ready.

5. Make them your own.

You can eat them as is or dress them up. I love them by themselves, but sometimes I need to kick it up a notch. Find your favorite add-ins and keep them on hand to turn scrambled eggs into a superquick gourmet breakfast. Here are some ideas to get you started . . .

Parmesan and pepper

Herbs

Cheese, cheese, and more cheese

Ham, jamón, prosciutto . . .

Caviar and crème fraîche

Artichokes

Truffles

Smoked salmon and dill

Olives and feta

Avocado

Caramelized onions

Tomatoes (fresh, raw, roasted, sun-dried . . .)

Baked Egg with Mushrooms and Spinach

Ditch the cereal, drop the frozen waffles, and, for goodness' sake, put down that Lender's bagel! Instead, pick up a ramekin and preheat the oven. The little ceramic vessels are perfect for housing eggs, meat, cheese, and vegetables and then tossing in the oven. What emerges ten minutes later is a perfectly cooked egg—whites soft but firm, yolk gloriously runny—surrounded by a tasty and filling supporting cast.

Serves: 4 / Prep time: 7 minutes / Cook time: 10 minutes

ALL YOU'LL NEED:

1 tablespoon olive oil

1 small onion, chopped

2 cups sliced mushrooms

4 slices Canadian bacon or deli ham, cut into thin strips

½ (10-ounce) bag frozen spinach, thawed

½ (7-ounce) can roasted green chiles

Salt and freshly ground black pepper

Butter, for ramekins

4 large eggs

PUTTING IT TOGETHER:

1. Preheat the oven to 375°F.

2. Heat the oil in a large skillet set over medium heat. Add the onion and cook for about 3 minutes, until translucent. Add the mushrooms and cook for about 5 minutes, until lightly browned.

3. Stir in the bacon, spinach, and chiles and cook for a few minutes, until the spinach is heated through. If any water from the spinach accumulates in the pan, carefully drain. Season with salt and pepper.

4. Divide the mixture among four 6-ounce oven-safe ramekins that have been lightly greased with butter. Carefully crack an egg into each, making sure to keep the yolks intact. Place the ramekins in a baking dish and bake until the whites are just set but the yolks are still runny, about 10 minutes.

French Toast Stuffed with Strawberries

I know it sounds decadent, but done correctly, stuffing can actually be a nutritional boon. Here, it adds a dose of protein, fiber, and all the energy-boosting vitamins from fresh strawberries. Plus, it's simple enough to pull off on a weekday morning, mimosa in hand.

Serves: 4 / Prep time: 5 minutes / Cook time: 10 minutes

ALL YOU'LL NEED:

1 cup low-fat ricotta or cottage cheese

½ cup skim milk

2 cups strawberries, sliced

2 tablespoons honey

2 tablespoons sliced or chopped almonds

1 tablespoon butter

2 large eggs

1 cup milk

¼ teaspoon ground cinnamon

1 teaspoon vanilla extract

8 slices whole wheat bread

Powdered sugar or pure maple syrup (optional)

PUTTING IT TOGETHER:

1. Place the ricotta, skim milk, strawberries, honey, and almonds in a mixing bowl and stir gently to combine. Set aside.

2. Heat the butter in a large cast-iron skillet or nonstick pan over medium heat. Beat the eggs with the milk, cinnamon, and vanilla in a shallow dish. Working one slice at a time, place the bread in the egg mixture, turning it over once to thoroughly coat, then add it directly to the hot pan.

3. Repeat until the pan is full.

4. Cook each slice for 2 to 3 minutes per side, until a golden brown crust is formed. Remove from the pan. Divide the strawberry mixture among four slices of the toast, spreading to evenly coat. Top each with another slice to make a sandwich, then slice on the diagonal to create two equal triangles. Serve with a shake of powdered sugar or a drizzle of maple syrup, if you prefer.

Eggs in Purgatory

It was a long night, and you feel every last drop of it when your feet hit the floor the next morning. Your head is pounding, your stomach is stirring, your body needs nourishment. Not a pile of greasy potatoes, but real food: protein, good carbs, a bit of healthy fat. But not just nutrients–flavors, too: spicy, sweet, creamy, salty. That's where these eggs come into play. They offer layers of intense flavors built around some of the healthiest ingredients in the pantry (tomatoes, garlic, whole grains). I like to call this my Hangover Helper.

Serves: 4 / Cook time: 27 minutes

ALL YOU'LL NEED:

½ cup uncooked farro or barley

1 ½ teaspoons olive oil

2 ounces pancetta or bacon, diced

½ medium-size onion, diced

2 cloves garlic, minced

½ teaspoon red pepper flakes

1 (28-ounce) can crushed tomatoes

Salt and freshly ground black pepper

8 large eggs

PUTTING IT TOGETHER:

1. Bring a pot of water to a boil over high heat. Add the farro and cook for about 20 minutes, until just tender. Drain.

2. While the grains cook, heat the olive oil in the largest cast-iron skillet or sauté pan you have. Cook the pancetta until lightly browned, then add the onion, garlic, and red pepper flakes and cook for about 3 minutes, until the onion is softened. Stir in the tomatoes and the farro and simmer for 5 minutes, until slightly reduced. Season with salt and black pepper.

3. Use the back of a large serving spoon to make eight small wells in the sauce. Crack an egg into each well. Cook over low heat for about 7 minutes, until the whites set but the yolks are still runny. You can use your fork to break up the whites so they cook more quickly.

4. Serve with whole wheat toast for scooping up the sauce.

LUNCH

As with gold diggers and professional golfers, lunch is all about the greens. It's the only meal of the day when eating a salad is acceptably naughty. And being strict about lunch gives you the nutritional confidence to let dinner happen as it may, whether it's chateaubriand for two at a white-linen restaurant, or a dozen canapés at a cocktail party, or a large popcorn at a movie theater.

Don't get me wrong: Lunch isn't about watching your calories. It's about packing as many nutrients into your body as you possibly can. Think of it as your daily paycheck–you're loading your savings account with healthy stuff, just in case you wind up blowing through your nutritional credit limit at dinner. The rules here are lots of green things as well as some healthy fats (a little fat makes the nutrients in produce more bioavailable), and not too many carbs. Lunchtime carbs tend to be the empty, sandwich-wrapping type. Save room for bread and pasta at dinner–not to mention dessert!

Caprese Tomato Towers

This classic Italian tomato salad from Capri is a study in simplicity: sweet, acidic tomatoes contrasted with creamy mozzarella slabs and the bright herbal bite of fresh basil. Why pay good money for such a simple pleasure you can make yourself only to let a restaurant screw it up with cheap parlor tricks? Make this one of your go-to summer salads.

Serves: 4 / Prep time: 10 minutes

ALL YOU'LL NEED:

4 medium-size tomatoes (preferably different colors of heirloom tomatoes)

6 ounces fresh mozzarella cheese (bonus points for burrata!)

16 large fresh basil leaves

Salt and freshly ground black pepper

1 tablespoon olive oil

½ teaspoon balsamic vinegar

PUTTING IT TOGETHER:

1. Slice the tomatoes into thick slices (each tomato should yield four or five slices). Slice the cheese into slightly thinner disks. There should be an equal number of tomato and cheese slices.

2. Place a tomato in the center of small salad plate.

3. Top with a mozzarella slice and a single basil leaf. Repeat until you've used up a quarter of the tomatoes, cheese, and basil (if you really want to nail this, salt and pepper each individual layer). If using different color tomatoes, alternate the slices throughout. Repeat on three additional small plates with the rest of the tomatoes, cheese, and basil, making four towers in all. Drizzle each tower with a bit of olive oil and balsamic and season again with salt and pepper.

Naughty Tip

This salad is probably not worth making
in the winter, when lifeless tomatoes are flown in from below
the equator. Come summer, though, when local tomatoes
are abundant, there's nothing better to eat.
Break out of the beefsteak box and explore the depth and
variety of heirloom tomatoes now available.
Each shape and color offers different levels of
sweetness and acidity, and even just sliced and salted,
make for an amazing salad.

Poached Egg over Frisée Salad with Bacon Dressing

There is something naughty about a poached egg, even though it's a healthy food. Adding in a little bacon ups the no-no quotient.

Serves: 1–2 / Cook time: 12 minutes

ALL YOU'LL NEED:

2 large eggs

White vinegar

2 strips bacon, chopped

1 head of frisée lettuce

Any other lettuce or greens you have on hand

Sliced bread (anything from a nice whole wheat to a rustic bread works here)

2 teaspoons mustard

1 ½ tablespoons red wine vinegar

2 teaspoons brown sugar

Salt and freshly ground black pepper

Before you start!
Tips for perfect poached eggs

Prep everything before you start;
poached eggs cook quickly and they
taste best served immediately.

Get the freshest eggs you can
(usually there is a 3-digit number on every
egg carton that corresponds to
the day those eggs were packaged).

PUTTING IT TOGETHER:

1. Crack each egg into a ramekin so you can help it into the water very gently.

2. Start by putting a wide, shallow pot filled two thirds of the way with water on medium heat. When the water is bubbling but not boiling–meaning you can see a few bubbles but they're not rising to the top or forming very quickly–add a dash of white vinegar. The vinegar helps the white stay together–if you are using a farm-fresh egg, the whites naturally stay together. With a supermarket egg, I think the vinegar is a nice insurance policy to help get a pretty egg!

3. Using a spoon or spatula, create a small whirlpool. Gently add an egg to the swirling water: just bring the ramekin to the water and softly pour the egg in.

4. Set a timer for 3 minutes. You can play around with time, but 3 minutes works for me. Because I set the timer after I have the egg in the water and then scoop it out after I hear the timer, it's probably in there closer to 3 ½ minutes, but it makes for a delicious egg.

5. Using a wide spoon, scoop out the egg and drain it on a thick paper towel, or if you have a slotted spoon, just let the water drain for a few seconds. Repeat with the second egg.

6. While the eggs cook, in a skillet on medium heat let the bacon cook down until browned, 2 to 4 minutes. Once the bacon is cooked through, take it off the heat and allow it to cool for a few minutes. If it's very fatty, drain some of the fat, but you should still have a tablespoon or so of fat in the pan. You are using it instead of oil, so you want to keep enough to make a dressing.

7. While the bacon cooks and cools, rinse the frisée and other greens thoroughly and separate the leaves. Pat them dry.

8. Toast your bread.

9. Put the bacon back on a very low heat. Add the mustard to the pan and stir well; add the red wine vinegar and the sugar and whisk until incorporated. Add salt and pepper to taste. Remove from the heat and allow to cool.

10. Quickly toss the lettuce in the bacon dressing and plate. Put your toast down on the salad and slide your eggs onto the toast.

Split Pea Soup

Split peas rank up there as one of the heroes of the health-food world, boasting deep reserves of fiber, B vitamins, and dozens of other vital nutrients. But despite their reputation as a straitlaced superfood, something magical happens to split peas when combined with a bit of smoky ham and a long, slow simmer. Slowly they begin to break down, commingling with the ham and the other vegetables to create a thick, creamy broth that could warm even the most frigid soul on a long winter day.

Serves: 6 / Prep time: 10 minutes / Cook time: 40 minutes

ALL YOU'LL NEED:

1 teaspoon olive oil

2 ribs celery, diced

1 small onion, diced

2 medium-size carrots, peeled and diced

2 cloves garlic, minced

10 cups water or low-sodium chicken or vegetable stock

2 medium-size red potatoes, peeled and diced

1 smoked ham hock

1 cup split peas

2 bay leaves

Salt and freshly ground black pepper

Tabasco (optional)

PUTTING IT TOGETHER:

1. Heat the olive oil in a large saucepan or pot over medium heat. Add the celery, onion, carrots, and garlic and sauté for about 5 minutes, until the vegetables are soft. Add the water, potatoes, ham hock, split peas, and bay leaves.

2. Turn the heat down to low and simmer for about 40 minutes, until the peas have turned very soft and begin to lose their shape, leaving you with a thick soup. (Thin with more water or stock if you prefer a thinner consistency.)

3. Remove the ham hock, shred the meat clinging to the bone, and add back to the soup. Discard the bay leaves. Season to taste with salt and pepper, plus a few shakes of Tabasco, if you like.

Avocado Toast with Red Pepper Flakes

I used guacamole as my inspiration for this one. Sometimes I just want to eat a whole bowl. This way, it's part of a meal.

Serves: 1 / Cook time: 6 minutes

ALL YOU'LL NEED:

½ avocado

1 bakery-fresh whole-grain baguette cut at a steep angle so there's enough room for all the toppings

⅛ teaspoon red pepper flakes

Maldon salt

1 teaspoon extra-virgin olive oil

Sprigs of fresh cilantro

1 wedge of lime

PUTTING IT TOGETHER:

1. Cut the avo open, stab the pit with a knife, and pull it out. *Ahhh, cathartic!* Cut the flesh (while it's in the skin) into very thin slices.
2. Toast the bread to your desired color.
3. Scoop the avocado from the skin (making sure to get the darker green flesh right along the peel), and gently fan evenly onto the toast.
4. Sprinkle with the red pepper flakes.
5. Take a pinch of Maldon. Crunch it between your fingers for finer flakes, and sprinkle evenly on the toast.
6. Drizzle the olive oil lightly over the avocado.
7. Finely mince the cilantro leaves and sprinkle over the toast.
8. Finally, squeeze a wedge of lime over the whole thing, and enjoy.

Quinoa Taboulé Salad

I have a Le Pain Quotidien a block away from me, and became addicted to this cleansing salad for a month straight–and then realized I can make it at home, using this official recipe. I love that the chain's founder, Alain Coumont, started Le Pain because he lived in Brussels and missed the salty bread of his childhood. Come to think of it, this lunch would go great with a hunk of Hazelnut Flûte.

Serves: 2 / Prep time: 10 minutes / Cook time: 30 minutes

ALL YOU'LL NEED FOR THE QUINOA TABOULÉ

- 1 cups cooked quinoa
- 1 medium-size beet, julienned
- 1 cup fresh parsley, chopped
- 4 fresh mint leaves, chopped
- 2 teaspoons dried currants
- 2 tablespoons freshly squeezed lemon juice
- 1 tablespoon extra-virgin olive oil
- Salt and freshly ground black pepper

ALL YOU'LL NEED FOR THE SALAD:

- 5 ounces arugula
- ½ cup canned or cooked chickpeas, drained and rinsed
- 1 ½ teaspoons extra-virgin olive oil
- 1 tablespoon freshly squeezed lemon juice
- ½ avocado, sliced
- Lemon wedges, for garnish

PUTTING IT TOGETHER:

1. Begin by preparing the quinoa taboulé. In a medium-size bowl, mix the cooked quinoa, beet, parsley, mint, and currants. Add the lemon juice, olive oil, and salt and pepper to taste until fully incorporated.

2. Next, make the salad: Place the arugula and chickpeas in a mixing bowl and drizzle with the olive oil and lemon juice. Season with salt and pepper, toss, and pile in the center of two plates.

3. Finally, measure 1 cup of quinoa taboulé for each serving and place loosely on top of the greens. Garnish with sliced avocado and lemon wedges, and voilà!

Grilled Ratatouille Salad

This is by no means a traditional ratatouille; it merely takes inspiration from the variety of vegetables that make up the ancient peasant dish from France. Nor does this recipe require every vegetable listed below, nor should it be confined to these ingredients. Don't have squash? No problem. Love tomatoes? Toss them directly onto the grill. That's the whole point of cooking: *You are in control.*

Serves: 4 / Cook time: 10 minutes

ALL YOU'LL NEED:

1 large red onion, cut into ¼-inch-thick slices

1 red bell pepper, quartered, stemmed, and seeded

1 medium-size eggplant, cut into ¼-inch-thick planks

1 large portobello mushroom cap, cut into ¼-inch-thick slices

1 large zucchini, cut into ¼-inch-thick planks

2 medium-size yellow squash, cut into ¼-inch-thick planks

12 to 16 asparagus stalks, woody ends removed

4 tablespoons olive oil

Salt and freshly ground black pepper

1 tablespoon prepared pesto

2 tablespoons red wine vinegar

2 tablespoons pine nuts, toasted

¼ cup grated Parmesan cheese

PUTTING IT TOGETHER:

1. Preheat a grill. Toss the vegetables with 2 tablespoons of the olive oil and generously season with salt and pepper. Grill the vegetables until cooked through and lightly charred, removing each individually when it has reached this stage. Some vegetables (like the onion and pepper) will take longer than others (like the asparagus and squash).

2. Combine the pesto and vinegar in a small bowl, then slowly drizzle in the remaining 2 tablespoons of olive oil. Cut the red pepper into thin slices, then toss all the vegetables with the vinaigrette, pine nuts, and Parmesan.

Avocado Dressing

The Naughty Girl eats salads, but only when she's craving one and only when it's well dressed and tastes delish. No sad side salads with dressing on the side for her! This dressing is packed with nutrients and whole ingredients AND it tastes way better than bottled ranch or creamy dressings. It is satisfying and makes even crudités feel decadent.

Serves: 1–2 / Prep/cook time: 5 minutes

ALL YOU'LL NEED:

½ avocado

1 ½ tablespoons olive oil

Juice of 1 lime

1 ½ teaspoons cider vinegar

Handful of herbs (I recommend a few leaves of mint and parsley)

Salt and freshly ground black pepper

PUTTING IT TOGETHER:

1. In a food processor, blender, or even by hand, combine the avocado with the olive oil, lime juice, cider vinegar, and herbs. Pulse a few times and add salt and pepper to taste.

2. I prefer to leave this dressing on the creamier side, but feel free to thin it with a little more lime juice and/or a few teaspoons of water.

PALATE CLEANSER

(INTER-COURSE)

Champagne Gelée

Why is this one Naughty? It's champagne! And it takes about five minutes in the kitchen to make it and then the fridge does most of the work for you. It's the perfect use for leftover bubbly (if the Naughty Girl ever has leftover bubbly) and it's the kind of treat that feels naughty even though it's quite nice.

Like many of the recipes to come–including the Roast Chicken, Rosé Popsicles and Caramelized Bacon Popcorn–this one's created by my friend Yasmina Jacobs of Eat Make Celebrate (eatmakecelebrate.com), the deliciously Naughty online resource for the modern woman.

Serves: 2 / Cook time: 5 minutes / Refrigeration time: 1 hour

ALL YOU'LL NEED:

1 cup elderflower cordial

½ cup very cold water

2 (¼-ounce) packets unflavored gelatin

1 ½ cups champagne

Raspberries or fruit slice, for garnish (optional)

PUTTING IT TOGETHER:

1. In a small saucepan, heat the elderflower cordial. It should be hot but not boiling.
2. Whisk the gelatin into the cold water. After whisking for a few seconds, pour in the hot elderflower cordial and continue to whisk for another 30 seconds or so, until the gelatin is completely dissolved.
3. Whisk in the champagne.
4. Transfer the mixture to a measuring cup or something that will make it easy to pour. Pour the mixture into disposable champagne coupes or small glasses.
5. Add raspberries or any other garnish to your glasses before refrigerating them for at least an hour.

SNACKTIME

The rule of snacking is simple: Put the stuff that's good for you out in the open. Hide the stuff that's bad for you deep in the cabinet. And make sure your snack has some protein, some healthy fat, and some fiber– or at least two of the three. Some things I rely on:

- Kale chips. Just drizzle a tablespoon of olive oil on kale leaves and bake at 250°F for 10 minutes. Season with some sea salt, garlic flakes, whatever's at hand.

- An apple, sliced up, smeared with peanut butter.

- A nice chunk of dark chocolate, similarly smeared.

- Or try this amazing snack to upgrade your Netflix nights.

Caramelized Bacon Popcorn

I feel bad for popcorn. When it's classified as a diet food, it's usually flavorless (not even salted!) and when it's served at the movies, it's half burnt and eaten mindlessly in the dark. Popcorn can and should be so much more. This is the ultimate movie night snack but it's also great as a party appetizer or sweet and savory treat.

Serves: 2 / Cook time: 7 minutes

ALL YOU'LL NEED

4 to 8 strips bacon

½ cup popcorn kernels

Vegetable oil (optional)

¼ cup honey

¼ cup granulated sugar

¼ cup brown sugar

1 teaspoon baking soda

Salt

PUTTING IT TOGETHER:

1. Chop the bacon into small chunks and brown it in a large, heavy, lidded pot.

2. Once the bacon is cooked, take it out of the pot, leaving behind any bacon drippings. Add the popcorn kernels to the pot–if you don't have much visible bacon grease, add a teaspoon of vegetable oil to the pot. Turn the heat up, and within a couple of minutes, you'll hear the popcorn start to pop. Shake the pot a few times to rotate the popcorn so you don't wind up with any burnt pieces or unpopped kernels.

3. Once you hear the popcorn slow down and one kernel or none is popping every second, take the popcorn off the heat.

4. To make the caramel, combine the honey, granulated sugar, and brown sugar in a saucepan and heat over low to medium heat for about 4 minutes, or until the mixture starts to bubble.

5. Take the sugar mixture off the heat and add the baking soda. Whisk in the baking soda for a few seconds and then crumble and add the bacon.

6. As soon as the bacon is incorporated into the caramel, pour it over the popcorn. Toss the popcorn making sure all the kernels are coated evenly.

7. Spread out the popcorn on a baking sheet lined with parchment paper, and sprinkle it with salt to taste.

DINNER

By the time dinner comes around, I feel like I've been behaving healthfully all day, and I'm ready for some naughtiness. On nights when you're feeling extra industrious–or just want to assert your feminine kitchen mystique for the entertainment of a fine young gentleman–these recipes are simple, healthy, and delicious–only the pizza takes time, and that's because it's authentically Italian. But they shouldn't stop you from answering the bell when a proper cocktail party calls.

Brick Lane Curry

Such is the food world we live in that even a simple vegetable stir-fry at a restaurant packs nearly 1,000 calories and a day's worth of sodium. It's a simple, unsuspecting dish that underscores just how vulnerable we are every time we decide to eat out. This Indian-style curry takes no more than 25 minutes to prepare, yet it will taste like it's been simmering away all day. The balance of the creamy coconut milk, the sweet cubes of squash, and the subtle heat of the curry powder could make the most dedicated meat eater forget she was eating only vegetables.

ALL YOU'LL NEED:

½ tablespoon canola oil

1 medium-size onion, diced

½ tablespoon minced fresh ginger

2 cups peeled, seeded, and cubed butternut squash

1 head cauliflower, cut into florets

1 (14- to 16-ounce) can garbanzo beans (a.k.a. chickpeas), drained

1 jalapeño pepper, minced

1 tablespoon yellow curry powder

1 (14-ounce) can diced tomatoes

1 (14-ounce) can light coconut milk

Juice of 1 lime

Salt and freshly ground black pepper

Chopped fresh cilantro

PUTTING IT TOGETHER:

1. Heat the oil in a large sauté pan or pot over medium heat. Add the onion and ginger and cook for about 2 minutes, until the onion is soft and translucent. Add the squash, cauliflower, garbanzos, jalapeño, and curry powder. Cook for 2 minutes, until the curry powder is fragrant and coats the vegetables evenly. Stir in the tomatoes and coconut milk and lower the heat to low.

2. Simmer for 15 to 20 minutes, until the vegetables are tender. Add the lime juice and season with salt and black pepper. Serve garnished with the chopped cilantro.

The Roast Chicken

There is something both decadent and homey about a roast chicken. You can feel like a domestic goddess out of a Norman Rockwell painting with minimal effort.

ALL YOU'LL NEED:

1 (4- to 6-pound) chicken

1 tablespoon kosher salt

1 teaspoon freshly ground black pepper

4 to 8 tablespoons (½ to 1 stick) unsalted butter, at room temperature

1 citrus fruit (Lemon is classic but oranges, tangerines, and limes are all delicious.)

Fresh herbs, like thyme, rosemary, or sage (optional)

Garlic, crushed (optional)

1 onion

PUTTING IT TOGETHER:

12 to 48 hours ahead

1. Dry brine the chicken: It may seem crazy to prep up this far ahead, but this step takes a just a few minutes and makes a world of difference! Dry brining is basically just putting a salt rub on the chicken. Without getting into the technicalities of poultry science, the salt helps the chicken retain moisture and is the foolproof way to get a deliciously juicy and tender bird.

2. Rinse the chicken and pat it dry (inside and out). Then, use your hands to sprinkle the salt all over the bird. A good ratio is about 1 tablespoon of salt to every 4 pounds of chicken. Once you've sprinkled the outside, make sure to get some salt in the cavity and use your fingers to get it all over the interior of the bird. You may not need all the salt; the goal is just to make sure you get some all over the chicken.

If you are a day (24 hours or less) out from cooking the bird, just place the salted chicken in the fridge uncovered. This will help dry out the skin, creating the perfect conditions for crispy skin. If you are more than 24 hours away from cooking it, loosely wrap it in plastic wrap, place it in the fridge, and uncover it a few hours before cooking time.

2 hours before serving

1. Preheat the oven to 375°F.

2. Take the chicken out of the fridge and pat it dry with a paper towel, wiping away any excess salt or excess moisture. Place the chicken in a roasting pan.

3. Mix the butter with the pepper and the zest of whatever citrus fruit you are using (reserve the whole fruit). For extra flavor, add any fresh herbs you have on hand and crushed garlic.

   Use your hands to loosen the chicken skin and spread some butter under the skin. Rub the rest of the butter all over the surface of the chicken.

   Chop the lemon and onion into quarters and place them in the cavity.

4. Roast for about 12 minutes per pound. With a 4- to 6-pound chicken, this should take anywhere from 50 to 75 minutes. Check on it halfway through your estimated cooking time. If the skin is browning too fast, add a little foil tent to protect the extra browned parts. You will know it's ready when the bird is golden brown and a meat thermometer reads 160°F. Let the chicken rest for at least 20 minutes before serving.

Classic Chicken Parm

This comfort classic is always a hit—and it should be in every Naughty Girl's arsenal.

ALL YOU'LL NEED:

4 boneless skinless chicken breast halves

½ cup all-purpose flour

2 large eggs

1 cup bread crumbs (Panko bread crumbs are my favorite.)

Salt and freshly ground black pepper

¾ cup Parmesan cheese

Olive oil

1 to 2 cups tomato sauce

¾ cup cubed or shredded mozzarella cheese

Other shredded melty cheese, like Gruyère or Cheddar (optional)

Basil, parsley, or other fresh herbs (optional)

PUTTING IT TOGETHER:

1. One at a time, place a chicken breast in a resealable plastic bag (or sandwich them in plastic wrap) and pound them out. If you don't have a meat pounder, a rolling pin or even an unopened bottle of wine will do. Pound and roll them out until they are ¼ to ½ inch thick.

2. Set out three plates. Place the flour in the first one, whisk the eggs in the second, and place the bread crumbs in the third. Add salt and pepper and ¼ cup of the Parmesan to the bread crumbs, and mix to combine.

3. Working with one chicken breast at a time, place the chicken in the flour—it should be lightly coated in flour on both sides. Next, dip into the eggs; again a light coating will do. Last, press it into the bread crumb mixture to make sure the whole breast has a nice, even layer of breading. Repeat until all four chicken breasts are coated.

4. Preheat the oven to 400°F.

5. Meanwhile, drizzle a little olive oil into a skillet, enough to visibly coat the bottom. Place over medium heat and give the oil a minute or so to heat up. Working in batches, brown the chicken. Depending on the

thickness and size, this should take about 2 minutes on each side. They don't have to be completely cooked through–that will happen in the oven.

6. Layer about one third of the tomato sauce into a casserole or baking dish. Place the browned chicken cutlets on top of the sauce.

7. Toss the remaining Parmesan together with the mozzarella and other cheese you have on hand. Sprinkle about a third of the cheese mixture over the chicken, followed by the rest of the tomato sauce, and then top with the remaining cheese mixture.

8. Bake for 20 to 30 minutes, or until the cheese is golden brown and bubbly. Serve with a little freshly grated Parmesan and chopped fresh herbs.

Lemon-Stuffed Mediterranean Sea Bass Wrapped In Foil

This dish whisks me away to the Mediterranean even before the first bite. They serve it on Mojito Island.

Serves: 1 or more / Prep time: 10 minutes / Cook time: 35 minutes

ALL YOU'LL NEED:

1 small branzino per person, butterflied and boned

6 lemons (or so)

Fresh thyme sprigs

Sweet vermouth

Sauvignon blanc

Kosher salt

Freshly ground black pepper

Olive oil

PUTTING IT TOGETHER:

1. Preheat the oven to 350°F. Line a baking pan with foil.

2. Rinse the fish and pat dry with paper towels, and open it with a knife.

3. Slice the lemons into thick slices and layer some in the bottom of the pan, then cover with some of the thyme sprigs.

4. Sprinkle a healthy amount of sweet vermouth over the lemons, and throw in a little sauvignon blanc as well since you're already drinking it.

5. Lay the fish down over the lemon slices and thyme.

6. Sprinkle with a tiny bit of salt, pepper, and olive oil, and stuff with the remaining lemon slices and thyme.

7. Close the fish and rub the skin generously with the salt and a sprinkle of olive oil.

8. Fold the foil over, creating a pocket, and bake on the center rack for 30 to 40 minutes, depending on the size of the fish. The skin will feel soft but the meat should be cooked through. Open it up to check.

9. For a crusted skin, open the foil and put the pan on the top rack for 5 minutes at 400°F. This may cause the skin to stick to the foil.

Naughty Cheat

Other fish can be used,
but the cooking time will need to be adjusted.
Lemongrass, garlic, parsley, cilantro,
or basil would also taste great! And instead of foil,
you can also use parchment paper
or put the fish on a grill.

The Caffeinated Coffee-Rubbed Steak

Coffee and steak might seem like an unlikely partnership, but the flavor of beef is actually heightened by the robust notes of java–plus, both are aphrodisiacs. This dish would be perfect with grilled vegetables and a side of black or pinto beans. Or heat up a few corn tortillas and pass them out so everyone can make their own little tacos. Either way, be sure to let the beef rest (even if it actually makes this ten-minute meal a twelve- or thirteen-minute meal); cut into it too early and all the still-hot juices will bleed onto your cutting board, instead of being reabsorbed by the meat.

Serves: 4 / Prep time: 7 minutes / Cook time: 20 minutes

ALL YOU'LL NEED:

½ tablespoon finely ground coffee or espresso

½ tablespoon chili powder

Salt and freshly ground black pepper

1 pound flank or skirt steak

Pico de Gallo

1 lime, quartered

PUTTING IT TOGETHER:

1. Preheat a grill, grill pan, or cast-iron skillet. Combine the coffee grounds with the chili powder, plus a few generous pinches of salt and pepper. Rub the spice mixture all over the steak. Cook the beef for 3 to 4 minutes per side, depending on its thickness, until slightly firm but still yielding.

2. Let the steak rest for at least 5 minutes, then slice thinly against the grain of the meat. Serve with a big scoop of pico de gallo and a wedge of lime.

Naughty Cheats

**Steak and coffee isn't the only
unconventional pairing
that yields surprisingly excellent results.
Try any of these tantalizing teams for
a jolt to your taste buds:**

——

**Watermelon and tomato,
topped with crumbled goat cheese and basil**

——

**Olive oil and ice cream,
with a pinch of coarse sea salt**

——

**Strawberries, balsamic vinegar,
and freshly ground black pepper**

——

**Peanut butter, banana, and bacon
between toasted bread
(the King would approve)**

——

Pizza with Arugula, Cherry Tomatoes, and Prosciutto

This pie is based on a pizza once eaten at a trattoria high above the ocean in the impossibly scenic village of Positano, which clings to the cliffs above Italy's Amalfi Coast. Although you'll have a tough time re-creating the setting, this combination of ingredients flirts with those magical flavors. The cherry tomatoes roast down into sweet little orbs of sauce, the prosciutto adds a salty punch, and the arugula, which wilts gently from the residual heat of the pizza, brings a fresh, peppery note to the pie. *Bellissima!*

Serves: 4 / Prep time: 20 minutes / Dough rise time: 2 days / Cook time: 8 minutes

ALL YOU'LL NEED FOR THE PIZZA SAUCE:

1 (28-ounce) can whole peeled tomatoes, drained

½ teaspoon salt

1 tablespoon olive oil

1 clove garlic, finely minced

ALL YOU'LL NEED FOR THE PIZZA DOUGH:

1 (½-ounce) package instant yeast

1 cup hot water

½ teaspoon salt

1 tablespoon sugar or honey

2 ½ cups white or whole wheat flour, plus more for kneading and rolling

TO ASSEMBLE AND BAKE:

1 cup Pizza Sauce

Pizza Dough, or be naughty and use a 12-ounce store-bought pizza dough, or large prebaked crust, such as Boboli

1 ½ cups shredded part-skim mozzarella cheese

2 cups cherry tomatoes

2 cups arugula

6 slices prosciutto, cut or torn into thin strips

Shaved or grated Parmesan cheese

PUTTING IT TOGETHER:

1. Make the sauce: Place all the sauce ingredients in a blender and puree for a few seconds, until the tomatoes have broken down but still retain some chunky texture. (Makes about 3 cups of sauce. Store the leftover sauce in the fridge for the next time.)

2. Make the dough: Combine the yeast with the hot water, salt, and sugar. Allow to sit for 10 minutes while the hot water activates the yeast.

3. Stir in the olive oil and flour, using a wooden spoon to incorporate. When the dough is no longer sticky, place on a cutting board, cover with more flour, and knead for 5 minutes.

4. Return the dough to the bowl, cover with plastic wrap, and let rise at room temperature for at least 90 minutes. (Keeps covered in the refrigerator for up to 2 days.)

5. Assemble and bake the pizza: Preheat the oven to 500°F. If you have a pizza stone, place it on the bottom rack of the oven.

6. Divide the dough into two equal pieces (unless you're using a prebaked crust). On a well-floured surface, use a rolling pin to work the dough into two thin circles, about 12 inches in diameter.

7. If you have a pizza stone, place one circle of dough on a pizza peel, cover with a light layer of the pizza sauce, then top with half of the mozzarella and cherry tomatoes. Slide directly onto the pizza stone and bake for about 8 minutes, until the edge of the dough is lightly browned. If you don't have a pizza stone, bake the pizza on a baking sheet instead.

8. Transfer the pizza to a cutting board and immediately top with half of the arugula (which will wilt lightly from the heat), half of the prosciutto, and a good measure of shaved or grated Parmesan. (If you have a large block of Parmesan, simply use a vegetable peeler to shave thin slices of cheese over the top.) Cut the pizza into six or eight slices.

9. Repeat with the other circle of dough and the remaining ingredients.

NAUGHTY DESSERTS

Move over breakfast, dessert is the most important*
meal of the day! It's the *grand finale* of every meal–
the cherry (and icing!) on the cake. The pleasure
of dessert lies in both the anticipation *and* the satisfaction. At restaurants I often survey the dessert menu
first since nothing whets my appetite more than saving
a sweet spot for sweets. This delayed dessert gratification
is the sexiest foodplay. No surprise then that
most Naughty Girls reach foodgasm right at the end.

When indulging in dessert, it's essential you let go,
dismiss any guilt and engage all your senses. This is
strictly not the time to fret over calories, worry about
workouts, fall food preggers, or discriminate against
the decadent. A carefree climate is most conducive to
confectionary climax! So keep calm and drool on…

*sensually speaking

Iced Berries Covered in Hot White Chocolate Sauce

This dessert is nicely naughty in every way: it's a breeze to make, berry good and sinfully decadent, it tickles the taste buds with hot and cold sensations and serving it is a feast for hungry eyes

Serves: 2 lovers / Prep time: 5 mins / Cook time: 6 mins

ALL YOU'LL NEED:

⅓ cup heavy cream

⅓ ounce white chocolate or a little more, for nibbling chefs

A shot or more of white rum (optional, but strongly advised)

1 cup mixed frozen berries (Most Naughty Girls have a bag of berries in the deep recesses of the freezer, from a former smoothie/health-kick phase.)

PUTTING IT TOGETHER:

1. Pour the cream into a small saucepan and break in the chocolate! Heat gently, stirring slowly, until the chocolate melts into a smooth sauce. Remove from the heat and add the rum.

2. Lay the frozen berries on a large plate.

3. Then (preferably with your date watching), do the honors of slowly pouring the hot creamy sauce all over your fruits. (Dirty mind!)

4. Share immediately, before the berries soften . . .

Chocolate Pudding with Olive Oil and Sea Salt

What really makes this pudding special is the final flourish. It might sound like a strange way to eat dessert, but the combination of chocolate, peppery olive oil, and crunchy little flakes of salt brings to mind a bag of chocolate-covered pretzels.

Serves: 4 / Prep time: 15 minutes / Refrigerator time: 2 hours

ALL YOU'LL NEED:

¼ cup sugar

2 tablespoons cornstarch

2 cups low-fat milk

1 tablespoon unsalted butter

4 ounces bittersweet or semisweet chocolate, chopped

(or ⅔ cup bittersweet chocolate chips)

1 teaspoon vanilla extract

Pinch of table salt

Olive oil

Coarse sea salt (like fleur de sel)

PUTTING IT TOGETHER:

1. Combine the sugar and cornstarch in a medium-size saucepan over low heat. Slowly add the milk, whisking to blend. Bring to a bare simmer, then stir in the butter, chocolate, vanilla, and table salt. Remove from the heat and continue stirring until the chocolate has melted uniformly. Pour into four small glasses or ramekins and place in the fridge for at least 2 hours.

2. Before serving, drizzle the puddings with a bit of olive oil and top each with a pinch of sea salt.

Naughty Cheats

**Three other ways to turn
this very good chocolate pudding
into something exceptional:**

———

S'MORES PUDDING
Line the bottom of the glasses with crushed graham crackers.
Top with marshmallows.

———

PB&C
Whip together equal parts milk and chunky peanut butter.
Divide among the glasses, then top with the pudding.

———

CHOCOLATE–COVERED STRAWBERRIES
Cover the bottom of each glass with sliced strawberries or
a heaping tablespoon of strawberry jam,
top with a thin layer of ricotta cheese,
then spoon in the pudding.

———

Molten Chocolate Cake

The idea of baking and frosting a multitiered chocolate cake is daunting for most, but these little self-contained parcels of joy are the lazy lady's cake, the type of dessert that makes a nonbaker feel like a pastry queen when they emerge from the oven, pregnant with a tide of melted chocolate. Crack the middle and watch the flood of lava flow freely onto your plate—and eventually into your eagerly awaiting mouth. Ahhh, that hits the P-Spot.

Serves: 4 / Prep time: 20 minutes / Cook time: 10 minutes

ALL YOU'LL NEED:

5 ounces bittersweet chocolate (at least 60% cacao), plus 4 chunks for the cake centers

2 tablespoons butter

2 large eggs

2 large egg yolks

¼ cup sugar

Pinch of salt

2 tablespoons all-purpose flour

1 teaspoon vanilla extract

½ tablespoon instant coffee or espresso (optional, but do it!)

PUTTING IT TOGETHER:

1. Preheat the oven to 425°F. Lightly butter four 6-ounce ramekins or custard cups.

2. Bring a few cups of water to a boil in a medium-size saucepan over low heat. Place a glass mixing bowl over the pan (but not touching the water) and add the chocolate and butter. Cook, stirring occasionally, until both the chocolate and butter have fully melted. Keep warm.

3. Use an electric mixer to beat the eggs, egg yolks, sugar, and salt until pale yellow and thick, about 5 minutes. Stir in the melted chocolate mixture, flour, vanilla, and instant coffee, if using.

4. Pour the mixture into the prepared ramekins. Stick one good chunk of chocolate in the center of each ramekin. Bake the cakes on the center

Affogato

Leave it to the Italians to come up with a two-ingredient dessert that satisfies as thoroughly as the most intricate cakes, pies, and pastries we normally find forced upon us at the end of a meal out. Affogato takes two traditional caps to a meal–ice cream and espresso or coffee–and combines them into one happy glass of gustatory joy. If you don't have an espresso machine, simply brew a brute-strength batch of coffee by using 1/4 cup of grounds and 1 cup of water. Use the best beans you can find, though, since the intensity of the coffee magnifies both flaws and finer points.

Serves 4 / Prep time: 6 minutes

ALL YOU'LL NEED:

2 cups vanilla ice cream or gelato   1 cup hot espresso

PUTTING IT TOGETHER:

1. Place one good scoop of vanilla ice cream or gelato in each of four small glasses (rocks glasses work nicely). Pour 1/4 cup of hot espresso over each scoop. Serve immediately.

Strawberry Shortcake with Balsamic Vinegar

Here, angel food cake picks up the smoke and char of the grill and is topped with strawberries soaked in balsamic vinegar and black pepper, an irresistible combination adored throughout northern Italy. Trust me, you'll be hooked.

Serves: 4 / Prep time: 12–18 minutes / Cook time: 5–10 minutes

ALL YOU'LL NEED:

2 cups sliced strawberries

¼ cup balsamic vinegar

Pinch of freshly ground black pepper

1 tablespoon butter (optional)

4 wedges angel food cake, each 1 inch thick

Whipped cream

PUTTING IT TOGETHER:

1. Mix the strawberries, vinegar, and pepper together and marinate for 10 to 15 minutes.

2. Heat a grill, stovetop grill pan, or nonstick sauté pan until hot. (If using the pan, add the butter; if grilling, omit the butter entirely.) Add the cake slices and cook until caramelized and toasted.

3. Transfer to four dessert plates. Top with the strawberries, their liquid, and a spoonful of whipped cream.

Bourbon Caramel Sauce

Why it's Naughty: two words, bourbon and caramel. This should be in every Naughty Girl's repertoire. It takes a few minutes to make and can be used to make ice cream taste dreamier or upgrade a store-bought dessert to impress company. No need to mention you made only the sauce.

Serves: 3 or more / Cook time: 15 minutes

ALL YOU'LL NEED:

1 cup sugar

⅓ cup water

⅓ cup heavy cream

1 teaspoon salt

1 teaspoon vanilla extract

1 to 2 tablespoons bourbon (rum, cognac, or brandy would work, too)

PUTTING IT TOGETHER:

1. Start by putting the sugar in a pan, then gently pour the water over the sugar so there are no dry patches. Heat, without stirring, over medium heat for 10 to 15 minutes, until the liquid turns an amber (caramel) color.

2. Take the pan off the heat and add the cream. Stir immediately to help incorporate the cream.

3. Add the salt, vanilla, and bourbon and place back on the heat for another minute or so. Stir for a few seconds until all the ingredients come together.

4. Pour into a bowl or dish and let the caramel cool for a few minutes before using. The sauce can be refrigerated and served cold or reheated before serving.

Rosé Popsicles

Sort of like sangria in a Popsicle. Easy, refreshing, summery, and a little bit naughty.

Serves: 4 or more / Prep time: 10 minutes / Freezer time: 2 hours

ALL YOU NEED:

1 cup fruit (I like to use berries like raspberries and strawberries; sliced peaches or cherries are great, too.)

3 cups rosé wine (3 cups is about 1 bottle)

⅓ cup Cointreau, Grand Marnier, brandy, triple sec, or other liquor

1 cup water

1 lemon or lime, sliced

PUTTING IT TOGETHER:

1. Slice or chop the fruit into bite-size pieces. If you are using small berries like raspberries, you can leave them whole.
2. In a large pitcher, stir together all the ingredients.
3. Once everything is combined, pour into Popsicle molds or even use a large ice cube tray in a pinch. Freeze for at least 2 hours.

Fruitylicious Crumble

Almost any fruit makes a delicious crumble–this is a basic guide to help you make a crumble out of whatever fruit is in your fridge–waste not, want not! Flavorful, seasonal, sweet, tart, and crunchy–and so simple, what more could you ask for? (Well, maybe a small scoop of ice cream to top it all off.)

Serves: 4 / Prep time: 20 minutes / Cook time: 30 minutes

ALL YOU'LL NEED FOR THE FRUIT FILLING:

3 to 5 cups fruit, measured after cutting (Almost any fruit works: peaches, plums, berries, pears, rhubarb, figs . . . you get the idea. Mix and match whatever is in season.)

¼ cup sugar, honey, or pure maple syrup (You can always add a bit more if the fruit is very tart.)

1 tablespoon cornstarch (Flour will work in a pinch.)

EXTRA FLAVORS:

Add a teaspoon of one or two extra flavors. Choose anything you like or that pairs well with the fruit you've chosen:

Lemon zest and/or lemon juice. I almost always use this.

Vanilla extract

Alcohol. Some of my favorite things to mix into cobblers include bourbon, orange liqueur, brandy, or flavored rum

Ground cinnamon

Herbs. Something savory like thyme can be a delicious surprise!

ALL YOU'LL NEED FOR THE CRUMBLE:

1 cup all-purpose flour

¼ cup sugar

1 teaspoon salt

8 tablespoons (1 stick) butter

One of the extra flavorings you added to the fruit (optional)

PUTTING IT TOGETHER:

1. Preheat the oven to 400°F.

2. Make the fruit filling: Cut any large fruit into slices or bite-size pieces. Toss the fruit with the sugar, the cornstarch, and any extra flavorings you'd like. Once everything is combined, place the fruit mixture in a baking dish.

3. Combine the crumble ingredients: the flour, sugar, salt, butter and any other flavors you want to include. Use your fingers to mix them together and break up the butter into pieces. It should look somewhat crumbly with visible pea-size pieces of butter throughout. Use your hands to sprinkle the topping onto the fruit.

4. Bake for 30 minutes, or until the top is browned and the fruit is cooked through.

Berry Wine Sorbet

Sorbet with wine. Wine sorbet. Need I say more?

Serves: 2 / Cook time: 15 minutes

ALL YOU NEED

1 cup water

⅔ cup sugar

2 cups berries (I like strawberries, blackberries or raspberries for this, but feel free to mix and match whatever fruit looks the best/ripest.)

1 ½ cups red wine

1 teaspoon vanilla extract

PUTTING IT TOGETHER:

1. In a small saucepan, combine the water and sugar. Heat, stirring, until the sugar is completely dissolved.

2. In a blender, combine all the ingredients, including the sugar syrup. Pulse until you reach a smooth, creamy consistency.

3. Place in an ice-cream maker and follow the manufacturer's instructions. If you don't have an ice-cream maker, pour the sorbet liquid into a dish, seal, and freeze for at least 3 hours. The sorbet won't be quite as creamy but it will be just as delicious. I recommend taking it out of the freezer about 5 minutes before serving.

The Naughty Nutrients

{Protein}

The Nutrient: Essential for maintaining muscle, protein burns fat because it takes a great deal of energy to digest it. It also helps you feel full longer.

How to Get Yours: Protein primarily means meats, like chicken, turkey, beef, fish, as well as eggs and dairy. I love shrimp cocktail or cooked prawns (hot or cold). Both are high in protein and low in fat. I sometimes just dunk cooked prawns into salsa or sauté frozen shrimp with a little garlic, chili powder, and black pepper as a high-protein snack or salad topper. Skip the tartar sauce and try horseradish or fresh lemon juice with your seafood.

I also like eggs for protein (cheap and easy). I never fry my eggs. I just add roughly 2 inches of boiling hot water to a skillet and cook my eggs sunny-side up that way. I also love a frittata–it's an easy way to sneak lots of good stuff into a meal like red peppers, spinach, mushrooms, and broccoli. I'll also add a little goat cheese to my frittata or sliver of Swiss cheese to my omelet.

{Healthy Fats}

The Nutrient: Healthy hair, skin, and nails come from healthy fats. So does that feeling of being sated and not needing to eat again. Monounsaturated fats, polyunsaturated fats, and omega-3 fatty acids should be part of your daily focus.

How to Get Yours: Include such things as olive oil and nuts. (It's a misconception that fat makes us fat; fat is essential for satiety and other body functions.) I get most of my healthy fats from avocado, sashimi (I love the fatty tuna and salmon), chia seeds, dark chocolate, coconut milk, cashew hemp milk, hummus, Greek yogurt, mozzarella, nuts, and peanut or almond butter. Some ideas for you to integrate them:

• Nothing is easier than mushing up half an avocado, adding a drop of lemon juice, salt, and red pepper flakes, and serving on a slice of wholegrain toast. (See my recipe on page 135.)

• Sprinkle nuts on salads for extra crunch and texture. Use flaked almonds, so it's easy to spread the nuts around the whole salad.

• Use hummus as dip but also as a spread on sandwiches.

• One of my favorite guilt-free desserts is creamy, full-fat Greek yogurt drizzled with honey and topped with flaked almonds or chopped walnuts (for crunch) and diced banana.

{Carbohydrates}

The Nutrient: Another scary word for people who diet, which is why I don't. Carbs are where we get the majority of our fiber and B vitamins.

How to Get Yours: I like quinoa, brown rice, oatmeal, and whole-grain bread. I also like pasta (but I get fresh, handmade pasta because quality counts!). Quinoa is my favorite go-to power food–my brain food, my beautiful-skin food, my energy food! It's my supergrain and also a complete protein (vegans listen up!), containing all nine essential amino acids. I like to cook my quinoa in chicken broth for added flavor. I make chicken and avocado quinoa salads, and I serve it as a side too, with meat and poultry.

{Fruits and Vegetables}

The Nutrient: Technically they belong to the carb family, but they get special mention because higher levels of fresh produce are associated with weight loss, regardless of calories.

How to Get Yours: I love all kinds of berries, which are relatively low in sugar and high in antioxidants. For veggies, I love yams, edamame, and homemade vegetable soups with beans and legumes. My favorite healthiest vegetable is kale. I love making kale chips–just drizzle a tablespoon of oil on kale leaves and bake at 250°F for 10 minutes. Season with sea salt, garlic flakes, red pepper, etc. Tip: You can use only a tablespoon of olive oil for a whole bunch of kale. How? Distribute the oil evenly by shaking the kale in a sealed plastic container. And my Green Goddess juice of kale, spinach, apple (or pear), ginger, celery and/or cucumber sorts me out when I've crossed too far over the line. I like to think of green juices as "health insurance coverage."

{Your Indulgence}

The Nutrient: Even if it is one of those weeks—the kind that start with a bloated feeling and are scheduled to end with a reunion or a wedding—making room for cheating is essential.

How to Get Yours: My favorite naughty food is pizza with a good bottle of red wine. Pizza should always be naughty, but food marketers do a lot of things to it to make it nasty (panfried dough, cheese-stuffed crusts, those creepy disks ringed with mini hot dogs). I make homemade pizza at least twice a week with a very thin crust, lots of heart-healthy marinara sauce (sometimes homemade and sometimes readymade) and a light sprinkling of finely grated, part-skim mozzarella cheese. Add fresh oregano, basil, and crushed garlic and choose healthier toppings like avocado, arugula, onions, chicken, mushrooms, and even spinach and broccoli to get a good balance of vegetables, carbs, and protein. It is infinitely satisfying and so quick and easy to make.

I drink red wine (pizza's best friend) at least every other day (for my heart health; wink, wink!), but I try to limit myself to two glasses a day, and always drink water in between. I firmly believe that life is too short to drink shit wine (TND Rule: quality trumps quantity), so when I do have vino, it's always special, it's worth it and très memorable! I count wine as a sweet treat (it's sugar, after all) and don't usually need dessert if I'm having a great cab with dinner.

8 FOODS BETTER THAN "FEMALE VIAGRA"

Is one bout of hot sex a month worth risking your health for?

That's the question we're facing with the FDA approval of Addyi, the new drug that boosts female libido. In studies, women who took the drug reported just one "extra sexually satisfying event" per month, and the FDA recommends you stop taking the "female Viagra" after eight weeks if you see no improvement. The drug works on the brain chemicals that affect mood and appetite, but the downside can be steep: drowsiness, nausea, and dizziness, and women who take it will be advised to refrain from alcohol and be wary of extremely low blood pressure and drug interactions.

Not. Naughty.

While women weigh the pros and cons, the editors of one of my favorite magazines, *Eat This, Not That!*, have uncovered new research that shows certain foods (all of them sinfully delicious) can have much the same effect—boosting mood, improving hormonal balance, and increasing blood flow—without the dizzying side effects. The next time you set aside an evening to channel Marvin Gaye, work some of these foods into your day.

Female Viagra Food #1
SPINACH

Come to think of it, Popeye and Olive Oyl *were* always chasing each other around. Eating spinach will not only help you get Victoria's Secret-ready—thanks to its appetite-suppressing compounds—but it will also put you in the mood by increasing blood flow below the belt. "Spinach is rich in magnesium, a mineral that decreases inflammation in blood vessels, increasing blood flow," explains Cassie Bjork, RD, LD, of Healthy Simple Life. "Increased blood flow drives blood to the extremities, which, like Viagra, can increase arousal and make sex more pleasurable," says psychotherapist and sex expert Tammy Nelson, PhD. "Women will find it is easier to have an orgasm, and men will find that erections come more naturally." And remember, "Having good sex is the best aphrodisiac," says Bjork. "It makes you want to have more sex!"

Female Viagra Food #2
GREEN TEA

The secret to a hotter nightlife starts with a hot cup of tea. Green tea is rich in compounds called catechins, which have been shown to blast away belly fat and speed the liver's capacity for turning fat into energy. But that's not all: Catechins also boost desire by promoting blood flow to your nether regions. "Catechins kill off free radicals that damage and inflame blood vessels, increasing their ability to transport blood," says Bjork, who recommends drinking four small cups a day. "Catechins also cause blood vessel cells to release nitric oxide, which increases the size of the blood vessels, leading to improved blood flow," she explains.

Female Viagra Food #3
PESTO

Pine nuts, one of the key ingredients in pesto sauce, are exceptionally high in zinc, and women with higher levels of zinc in their system have been shown to have a higher sex drive than those with lower levels.

Female Viagra Food #4
RED WINE

If you're looking for a way to simultaneously boost your libido and calm those predate jitters, pour yourself a glass of red. Women who drank one to two glasses had heightened sexual desire compared to ladies who didn't down any vino, a *Journal of Sexual Medicine* study found. (Just be sure to cut yourself off after your second glass; enjoying more than that didn't stimulate any further arousal, and knocking back too much can stop the show before it starts.) What makes the elixir so beneficial is a rich antioxidant profile that triggers nitric oxide production in the blood, which relaxes artery walls. As with many of the foods on this list, that increases blood flow down south.

Female Viagra Food #5
STEAKS AND BURGERS

If your crazy-busy schedule is to blame for your lack of libido, you're not alone. "One of the primary reasons couples stop having sex is because they're tired, fatigued and stressed. But sometimes, there's a biological component at play," says Nelson. One of the causes of fatigue in women is iron deficiency. The condition can sap energy, which may result in a low sex drive, Nelson explains. Bjork concurs, adding, "Iron deficiency is common and can result in feelings of exhaustion, weakness, and irritability, which doesn't make anyone feel like getting intimate."

Naughty Tip

**Bjork says remedying the situation
requires a two-part approach:
"If you think your diet lacks iron,
focus on eating more spinach,
grass-fed red meat
and liver, all foods rich in the nutrient.
Then, ensure sure your body is able
to utilize the iron," she says.
"Consuming probiotic-rich yogurt,
fatty fish and an
L-glutamine supplement can improve
gut health and help your body
to absorb iron more efficiently."**

Female Viagra Food #6
FATTY FISH

It's no secret that oily cold-water fish like wild salmon, sardines, and tuna are overflowing with omega-3 fatty acids, but here's something you may not know: The nutrient not only benefits your heart but also raises dopamine levels in the brain. This spike in dopamine improves circulation and blood flow, triggering arousal, Bjork and Nelson reveal. There's more: "Dopamine will make you feel more relaxed and connected to your partner, which makes sex more fun," adds Nelson.

Female Viagra Food #7
COFFEE

A recent survey discovered that the #1 spot for first dates is Starbucks. Looks like we've figured out why. In a recent study—albeit on animals—coffee consumption was found to make females more eager to engage in sex, and more likely to want it again after a brief rest. But studies show that men are more sensitive to caffeine than women are; guys begin to react within ten minutes of sipping joe. Since decaf also creates an enhanced level of alertness, a buzz-free bean might be the right pick-me-up for guys and dolls who want to avoid first-date jitters.

Female Viagra Food #8
DARK CHOCOLATE

Good news, chocolate lovers: Your go-to indulgence can help get you in the mood. Dark chocolate contains flavonoids that have been shown to reduce stress and relax blood vessels, sending blood to all the right regions—no Twinkie can claim that. Those same flavonoids can also help diminish body fat, which can boost your confidence in bed, making it easier to focus on the main attraction. My go-to bar is Lindt 85% Cocoa Excellence.

Step 9

CHILL THE EFF OUT

OLD RULE:
Downtime is for lazy people.

NAUGHTY WAY:
Sleep your way to the top.

PSSST! NAUGHTY GIRL: Do you want to
know the *simplest* way to lose weight, look like a billion bucks, and live a rich
and fulfilling life?

Anyone out there shaking her head no?

I heard the body- and life-changing advice at a TEDWomens conference
a few years ago. I'd recently moved to New York and was struggling with
my too-full-and-growing Big Apple agenda. Even deciding what to have for
breakfast seemed a task all too time-consuming. (Toast or oatmeal? A bagel?
Yogurt? Eggs? Fruit? . . .) For the first time in my life I had puffy bags under
my eyes; I felt bloated, heavy, off-balance. And despite eating as I had done
for years, my boyfriend jeans had started to feel like skinny jeans. I was sick
and tired of it. Or just sick and tired.

I can remember standing in the kitchen, having decided to make a quick slice of avocado toast before a morning of back-to-back-meetings, when I discovered I was out of bread. The tears welled up. *I really don't have time for this!* Thankfully my phone vibrated and distracted me from throwing a wobbly over avocado toast. It was a publicist friend with a last-minute invite:

"Have two passes for a TED talk this evening in DC. Come with?"

My schedule didn't allow for it.

I texted back.

"Pick me up at noon? Sounds amazing."

And it was. Only when we arrived did I learn the lecture was on productivity and happiness (how fitting!), and the speaker was Arianna Huffington—one of the most influential and successful women in media.

She shared a story about how she came to believe that proper R&R is the great key to success. It wasn't until she passed out at work one day, hit her head on her desk, broke her cheek, and needed stitches that she realized that prioritizing relaxation needs to be a foundational habit for any woman who wants to live a life of health and passion.

"It's time that women sleep their way to the top," she said.

I never forgot her advice. And I never will.

After the lecture, I couldn't wait to dive into research on the power of relaxation for the Naughty Diet.

. . . after a nap

. . . and a bubble bath

. . . and a glass of wine

. . . and an early night

I needed to stop *doing* and start *being*. I needed to chill the eff out.

How We Talk Ourselves into a Hot Mess

THINK ABOUT THE LAST TIME you ran into someone you hadn't seen in a while. I bet the conversation started just like this:

"Oh my God, hi! How are you?"

"Crazy busy. You?"

"Crazy!"

"Crazy busy" is the new "I'm fine." If we're not crazy busy, then something must be wrong. Maybe it's a post–Great Recession kneejerk response, a way of telling ourselves and others that we're fully engaged and fully employed. But each encounter reinforces the same suspicion: unless we're busy, we're worthless.

Or think about the last time someone called or texted you while you were sleeping.

"Did I wake you?"

"No, I'm up." Admitting that we were asleep–even late at night or early in the morning–is just too shameful, as if we were hopeless slackers for closing our eyes for a moment. When we're asleep, we're not busy. And when we're not busy . . . well, you know what that means. My life is full of strong, proud, accomplished women: There is nothing they can't do. Except, of course, doing nothing.

For so many women, being in a state of not doing is considered the ultimate luxury: an exotic flower that only blooms at luxurious five-star, adults-only hotel spa resorts. Peace of mind is the impossible dream. And thank God for Xanax.

Naughty News Flash: You don't have to travel to Tibet or pop pills to unplug, unwind, and find deep relaxation. It is, in fact, a native plant in your own backyard . . . try as you might to repeatedly uproot it. I'm here to help you cultivate the seeds of serenity. In your everyday life. While you breathe. While you eat. Or take a bath. Or wait for the subway.

Learning to relax means reasoning with your reason. It means cajoling your mind to let go of its grip. The crazy truth is that the harder we try to hold on–in an effort to control our health, weight, and lives–the more easily those things can pop out of our grasp. After all, the key to being in control is maximizing pleasure. And it's difficult to feel pleasure when you're tightly wound.

9 WAYS TO LOSE WEIGHT WHEN YOU'RE CRAZY BUSY

"Crazy busy." There's no escape from it. No matter who you ask—family, friends, colleagues, retirees, people in solitary confinement—everybody seems to be "crazy busy." You're crazy busy, too. Everyone from your mom to your college roommate to your boss expects immediate feedback to their latest e-mail, Instagram, or text message—while you're crazy busy sharing your own.

That's a lot of pressure. No wonder you don't feel you can find time to take care of yourself and finally get rid of that extra belly fat. Well, my friends at *Eat This, Not That!* discovered some good news: you don't need any extra time.

In Just 2 Seconds
ORDER A "COFFEE, BLACK."
A cup of coffee has nearly zero calories. A cup of coffee with cream and sugar has 80 calories. If you drink two cups a day, learning to take it black will save you 14 pounds in a year.

In Just 5 Seconds
TAKE A WHIFF.
Smelling fresh green apples, bananas, and pears can curb appetite and make sugary desserts less appealing, studies have shown.[1] The scientists suggest this is because the produce makes you subconsciously think about making healthier choices. If a fruit basket on your desk attracts too many flies, try a simpler idea, like a shea butter-based scented lotion, which will have the same effect.

In Just 15 Seconds
TAKE A CANDY DAYDREAM.
A recent study found that fantasizing about eating an entire packet of your favorite candy before indulging may cause you to eat less of it.[2] For the study,

researchers asked participants to imagine eating eight or eighty M&M's, and then invited them to help themselves to some of the candies as a "taste test." Those who imagined eating lots of M&M's actually ate the least.

In Just 60 Seconds
SCHEDULE A WORKOUT DATE.

It's hard to squeeze in a workout before meeting friends for drinks, so you blow off . . . the workout, of course. A better idea: Tell your bud to meet you at the gym. You can socialize, get fit, and still hit the bar afterward. This trick works with spouses, too: a recent *JAMA Internal Medicine* study of nearly four thousand couples found that people are more likely to stick to healthy habits like exercise when they team up with their partner.[3]

In Just 75 Seconds
NUKE FROZEN VEGGIES.

While frozen produce has a nutrient density that's often higher than fresh; canned foods don't hold up. A study in the *Journal of the Science of Food and Agriculture* found that for some vegetables, canning degraded as much as 95 percent of the vitamin C and damaged every B vitamin in the food.[4]

In Just 90 Seconds
TAKE YOUR OATMEAL HIGH-TECH.

Thank you, Nature Valley, for meeting us here in 2015 with your ingenious new Bistro Cups Oatmeal. It's a packet of dried oats, a sleeve filled with nuts and dried fruit, and a K-cup filled with flavoring. You put the dry ingredients in a mug, pop the K-cup in a Kureg, and hit Brew. According to a *Journal of the American College of Nutrition* study, hot oatmeal is more effective than cold cereal at reducing hunger.[5] (Don't have a Kureg? Quick Quaker Oats take only a minute to cook.)

In Just 100 Seconds
GET STONED . . . FRUIT.

New studies suggest that stone fruits—like plums, peaches, and nectarines—may help ward off belly fat, high cholesterol, and insulin resistance.[6] The belly-flattening properties of the fruit may come from powerful phenolic compounds that help modulate the expression of your fat genes. Eat one as a snack, or chop it up and toss it on your morning cereal or afternoon salad.

In Just 2 Minutes
PREGAME YOUR DINNER.

While it may sound counterintuitive, eating before going to a work dinner or happy hour can actually take off pounds. A series of studies out of Penn State found that noshing on an apple or a broth-based soup prior to sitting down to a restaurant meal can reduce total calorie intake by 20 percent.[7] With the average restaurant meal weighing in at 1,128 calories, saving 20 percent once a day could help you lose up to 23 pounds this year.

In Just 10 Minutes
SLOW-COOK A BEEF FEAST.

This is a great one for busy weekends: Heat 1 tablespoon of canola oil in a pan over high heat and brown a 3-pound chuck roast on all sides for about 10 minutes. In the meantime, slice some onions and mushrooms. When the meat's browned, throw it into a slow cooker and add the onions, mushrooms, 2 tablespoons of red wine vinegar, 1 tablespoon of Worcestershire sauce, some bay leaves, and a can of dark beer. Put it on low and go about your Sunday. Six hours later, you'll have an incredible dinner at the ready for just 345 calories per serving!

Adapted with permission from *Eat This, Not That!*

How to Chill

QUICK QUESTION: Why do we need "convenience food"?

Well, you'd need convenience food if eating were, in fact, inconvenient. If it were something to get out of the way because it interferes with what really matters to you in life.

Let's stop and think about that. If eating is essential to survival, and if the quality of what you eat–and the pleasure you derive–is essential to living healthfully, then what on earth is more important? What is it, exactly, that's being "inconvenienced" by your sitting down to enjoy a good meal? Or let me put it another way: Who decided that your health and happiness comes second?

If you're a doer, an achiever, a go-getter–oh hell, if you're just an average, everyday woman–then chances are you've got 101 people who need-you-right-now, and you're used to doing everything fast and furiously. Including, and especially, eating. So, maybe you nibble at your desk in between meetings, or grab a protein bar to eat in the car while racing to your next errand.

When you're zipping around like a boss lady on a million-dollar mission, your stress response is activated. Your heart rate speeds up, blood pressure increases, and your system is flooded by hormones that help to keep you alert–including cortisol and insulin, which have the very inconvenient side effects of making you crave sugar (even when you're full) and hold on to belly fat. (Is it any coincidence that *stressed* spelled backward is *desserts*?) Blood moves from the tummy to the brain to help you make quick, smart decisions. This is fight-or-flight mode–an evolutionary response geared to survival that's incredibly useful if you're running from a saber-toothed tiger, or haven't washed your hair for a week and happen to spot your very good-looking ex in the same line at the grocery store. Yikes, gotta go! Ain't nobody got time to digest Cheerios!

The same part of our brain that turns on stress also turns off digestion. And conversely, the part of the brain that turns on relaxation also turns on powerful slimming power. Maintaining a lean and sexy body, then, means keeping the relaxation switch in the on position.

Put Your Sexy on "Automatic"

THE MAGIC ENGINE that controls your stress-relax-stress response, and hence your ability to derive both pleasure and sustenance from food, is called the autonomic nervous system (ANS). The ANS is made up of two branches, the sympathetic and parasympathetic nervous systems, which work in tandem to tell your body when to metabolize food and when to shut things down. (Like when there's no food in your tummy to digest, or when you're running from a wild animal. Like your ex.)

If you're eating for pleasure, moving regularly, yet still struggling to lose weight, consider your stress levels. Is every decision you make based on how happy or unhappy a dozen other people will be with your choices? Does it take you longer to open an envelope than it does to eat a granola bar? Do you regularly boast to your co-workers about how little sleep you got last night? Do you spend your days with your jaw and bum cheeks clenched?

And the last time someone asked how you were, did you answer "crazy busy"?

If so, no amount of juicing or *SoulCycle* will get you closer to the body you want, physically or emotionally. That's because chronic stress decreases "thermic efficiency"–your ability to burn calories at rest. And what's one nasty form of chronic stress? Worrying about your weight. I'll put it to you this way: worrying about fat makes you fat.

There are many ways to build more relaxation into your life. The Naughty Diet prioritizes a handful: proper breathing, quality sleep, bubble baths, and, of course, oenotherapy, a.k.a. a glass of wine.

Inhale the Good Shit.
Exhale the Bullshit.

LEARNING TO BREATHE properly, deeply, and luxuriously is an effortless high. And much cheaper and cleaner than anything your doctor can prescribe. Few things are as satisfying as a gentle deep-breath dive into serenity–or as powerfully slimming.

You know by now I'm not a fan of calories. Counting them, clocking them, worrying about them–a total waste of time. Even typing the word causes my upper lip to curl. But for the purpose of explaining the weight-loss power of breathing, it's important to understand what a calorie actually is. A calorie is no more than a unit of energy, measured by the amount of time it takes something to burn. Everything has calories. A 100-calorie pack of almonds has between 80 and 120 calories (by law the labels can be off by 20%–one more reason to ignore them!). But even this page of paper you're reading has calories too (about 6). All of these calories need oxygen to burn. And because a fire feeds off oxygen, it follows that the greater your capacity to take in oxygen, the higher your calorie-burning potential. It's really that simple.

The digestive system is hungry for oxygen. The intestines in particular–the predominant site of nutrient absorption–extract large quantities of oxygen from the blood during the breakdown of a meal. The more we eat, the more the body wants us to breathe. If you start shallow breathing in a panic over the fat grams and flabby-arm consequences of what you just consumed, you're limiting your ability to burn calories and to extract nutrients.

You Are Now Breathing Manually

IN OUR CULTURE there is a lot more emphasis on inhaling than on exhaling. We associate a deep gulp of air with doing something useful, but we expel CO_2 with about as much passion as we use to toss out the garbage–always hurried, nose pinched. We receive almost no pleasure from relaxing our chest, clearing our airways, and sending forth a generous puff of carbon dioxide into the atmosphere. Even if it does promote photosynthesis.

Here's how to breathe away the pounds–properly:

1. **Open your mouth and gently sigh**, as if someone has just told you something really annoying. Like, you just showed up for your manicure appointment and your go-to girl is out sick. *Sigh.* As you do, let your shoulders and the muscles of your upper body relax, down, with the exhale. (If you're sitting, correct your posture. Sitting up straight makes for deeper, more luxurious breaths; more important, no one looks sexy when she slouches.)

2. Now close your mouth and pause for a few seconds.

3. Keep your mouth closed and inhale slowly through your nose by pushing your stomach out (don't do this in a crop top). When you've inhaled as much air as you can comfortably without feeling faint or looking weird (remember, you want to be able to do this in public restaurants), stop inhaling. And pause briefly.

4. Open your mouth. Exhale through your mouth letting your belly gently deflate like a balloon.

5. Pause briefly. Close your mouth, and repeat steps 1–5. Do this five times before a meal, snack, or to divert any panic attack.

Sleep Your Way to the Top

AT HER TEDWOMEN TALK, Arianna Huffington opened my eyes to the value of shutting them more. Before my trip to DC, I, like so many, was convinced that a lack of sleep was some sort of virility symbol. I once dated a guy who used to "operate" on just two to three hours of sleep. (I kept my own slovenly seven-hours-a-night habit to myself.) The relationship quickly burned out because he was always burned out–stuck in a perma-state of wired and tired. Sleep doesn't just help the body process food; it helps us process information. Stop sleeping, and you stop growing.

Even if you change nothing about your dietary habits, getting proper sleep–at least seven hours a night–can help you slim down. I've spent hours in the Pub (that's PubMed) reading up on the sleep-metabolism connection. Here are the highlights:

- During sleep your body secretes a large amount of growth hormone that tells your body how to break down fat for fuel. If you don't get enough sleep, your body just never gets the memo.

- Poor sleep decreases metabolic rate (the rate at which we burn calories) and increases cravings for sweets, carbs, and high-fat foods. It's the perfect storm for binge eating and rapid weight gain.

- Poor sleep lowers the level of leptin (the "I'm full" hormone) and increases production of ghrelin (the "Feed me!" hormone). You feel hungrier, even when the body should be sending signals that it's had enough, thank you.

- When you're sleep deprived, you snack more. One study found that when people slept for only five and a half hours, they ate normally at mealtimes, but consumed way more snacks![8] All between the hours of eleven p.m. and seven a.m.!

- One recent study reported that losing just thirty minutes of sleep per night increased the risk of obesity by 72 percent.[9]

- And when I asked women in my Naughty Survey how a lack of sleep affected their diet, 43 percent said they eat nasty, less nutritious food, 39 percent said they "eat more," and 41 percent said they feel "less in control of how and what I eat." Only 8 percent said they eat less. Only three ladies said they eat healthier food on less sleep!

Bottom line: Sleep more, and you'll gain more control over what you eat. Less junk, more pleasure.

Naughty Tip

No matter how much you love that one bra that makes you look perfectly perky day in and day out, no fabric touches you more than your bedsheets. And investing in top-quality linens is one of the greatest gifts you can give yourself. The more comfortable you are in bed—whether you're lounging, sleeping, or making love—the more relaxed you will feel and the more pleasure you will receive. There are many types of sheets. Egyptian cotton, grown only along the Egyptian section of the Nile River, is truly the Naughty Girl standard. The fabric has very long fibers that make a thinner thread, usually 200 count or more. The higher the thread count, the longer lasting and more luxurious.

8 WAYS TO LOSE WEIGHT WHILE YOU SLEEP

What's the best place in the world to lose weight?

The gym! say the muscle-bound personal trainers, raising their hands (but not really getting that high because their deltoids get in the way).

The (huff!) *track* (puff!) say the distance runners, bicyclists, triathletes, and other types trucking along with sweat in their eyes and numbers stuck on their chest.

The kitchen! say the nutritionists, dietitians, organic produce purveyors, and washed-up chefs slinging faux diet plans to the masses.

But they're all wrong. Because real, successful, sustainable weight loss comes from achieving excellence in a completely unexpected realm: the bedroom.

No, you can't lovemake your way to lean. But you can absolutely sleep your way to slender. In fact, no matter how many pounds you press, how many miles you log, how much kohlrabi you crunch, it won't get you anywhere near your weight-loss goals unless you're also getting enough quality sleep. A recent study found subpar sleep could undermine weight loss by as much as 55 percent![10] The good news is just a few simple tweaks to your p.m. routine can mean serious weight-loss success. So, open your eyes: here are eight science-backed suggestions to lose while you snooze.

1. **Tryp Your Sleep Switch.** Don't count sheep, eat lamb! (Or better yet, a bit of turkey.) Tryptophan, an amino acid found in most meats, has demonstrated powerful sleep-inducing effects. A recent study among insomniacs found that just ¼ gram—about what you'll find in a skinless chicken drumstick or 3 ounces of lean turkey meat—was enough to significantly increase hours of deep sleep.[11] And that can translate into

easy weight loss. Researchers from the University of Colorado found that dieters consumed 6 percent fewer calories when they got enough sleep.[12] For someone on a 2,000-calorie diet, that's 120 calories per day, which could amount to nearly a 1-pound weight loss in a month! The National Sleep Foundation suggests seven to eight hours of sleep for most adults.

2. **Set Strict Kitchen Hours.** Nighttime fasting—a.k.a. closing the kitchen early—may help you lose more weight, even if you eat more food throughout the day, according to a study in the journal *Cell Metabolism*.[13] Researchers put groups of mice on a high-fat, high-calorie diet for one hundred days. Half of them were allowed to nibble throughout the night and day on a healthy, controlled diet, while the others only had access to food for eight hours, but could eat whatever they wanted. The result of the sixteen-hour food ban? The fasting mice stayed lean, while the mice who noshed 'round the clock became obese—even though both groups consumed the same amount of calories!

3. **Shake Things Up.** Having a protein shake before hitting the sack may boost your metabolism, according to one Florida State University study.[14] Researchers found that men who consumed an evening snack that included 30 grams of either whey or casein protein had a higher resting metabolic rate the next morning than when eating nothing. Protein is more thermogenic than carbs or fat, meaning your body burns more calories digesting it.

4. **Make a Mint.** Certain scents can make your mouth water, and others can actually suppress your appetite. One study published in the *Journal of Neurological and Orthopaedic Medicine* found that people who sniffed peppermint every two hours lost an average of 5 pounds a month![15] Banana, green apple, and vanilla had similar effects. Consider burning a minty candle until you head to bed to fill the room with slimming smells. If you don't want to bother with blowing out candles before you turn down the covers, try adding a few drops of peppermint oil to your pillow.

5. **Let in the Cold.** A striking new study published in the journal *Diabetes* suggests that simply blasting the air conditioner or turning down the heat in winter may help us attack belly fat while we sleep.[16] Colder temperatures subtly enhance the effectiveness of our stores of brown fat—fat keeps you warm by helping you burn through the fat stored in your belly. Participants spent a few weeks sleeping in bedrooms with varying temperatures: a neutral 75 degrees, a cool 66 degrees, and a balmy 81 degrees. After four weeks of sleeping at 66 degrees, the subjects had almost doubled their volume of brown fat. (And yes, that means they lost belly fat.)

6. **Throw Out the Night Light.** Exposure to light at night doesn't just interrupt your chances of a great night's sleep, it may also result in weight gain according to a new study published in the *American Journal of Epidemiology.*[17] Study subjects who slept in the darkest rooms were 21 percent less likely to be obese than those sleeping in the lightest rooms.

7. **Get the Nighttime Blues.** There's a reason why McDonald's, Burger King, and Wendy's all have the same red-and-yellow theme colors. Those tones supposedly send us subliminal messages that help make us hungry. Does the same trick work at home? An experiment published in the interior design magazine *Contract* presented partygoers with three identical venues painted different colors: red, yellow, and blue. Participants reported the red and yellow rooms to be equally appetizing, but found the food in the blue room only half as appealing.[18]

8. **Hide the iPad.** Research suggests that the more electronics we bring into the bedroom, the fatter we get—especially among children. A study in the *Pediatric Obesity* journal found that kids who bask in the nighttime glow of a TV or computer don't get enough rest and suffer from poor lifestyle habits.[19] Researchers found that students with access to one electronic device were 1.47 times as likely to be overweight as kids with no devices in the bedroom. That increased to 2.57 times for kids with three devices. Leave your iPad in the living room.

When in Doubt, Take a Bath

EVEN OUT OF WATER, the Naughty Girl is wallowing in a luxurious bubble bath of her own sexy cells. Two thirds of the weight of the human body is a liquid that has roughly the same density and chemical composition as the beautiful briny sea. Skinny dipping in the privacy of your own home in the huge enameled seashell that is your bathtub lets you connect with your primordial self–a soothing remedy that I truly believe can improve everything from the disappearance of a lover to the appearance of cellulite. One study found that submerging in hot water can be as good for the heart as a slog on the *dreadmill*, as the hot temperature increases the volume of blood pumping to and from the organ.[20] And another study among diabetic patients who were required to soak in a hot tub for thirty minutes a day, six days a week, lost an average of 1 pound per week, which researchers attribute solely to soaking at the spa.[21]

There's an added benefit of making a naughty ritual of a regular wallow in the tub: you'll spend more time naked. The more often you practice the art of undressing when you're alone, the less anxious you'll be when you're not. And I'm not just talking about sex. Even dropping your sarong on Mojito Beach will be less of a *quick-sit-down-before-they-see!* moment. According to one survey, a majority of women spend less than ten minutes per day in the buff. And yet we angst about our naked selves constantly. Want to make peace with your thighs and feel hotter in a bikini? Run a bath, not a marathon! Whatever your want, worry, or doubt, a bath is the perfect naughty remedy.

Recipe for a Truly Decadent Bath

1 DO NOT DISTURB sign
1 bottle chilled bubbly (may substitute wine)
1 flute (or wineglass, as above)
1 large capful bubble bath (shower gel works just fine)
1 extra-large fluffy white towel (Four Seasons quality)

1 terry robe
1 hair tie
Scented candles (lavender for relaxation and grapefruit* if you're expecting
    company . . .)
Bath oils and/or salts (optional)
Relaxing spa music (optional, too)
Rose petals (OK, I'll stop now)

METHOD:
Draw bubble bath.
Turn off phone.
Eff all Guilt.
Soak for at least 20 minutes.

*Men cannot resist the scent of grapefruit. Want to spice things up with your man? Get a boyfriend?
Take the edge off a not-so-fun conversation with your husband? Douse yourself in grapefruit everything. Thank me later.

WINING IS WINNING

I like to relax with a glass of wine after a long glass of wine.
#NaughtyTweet

I WASN'T ALWAYS a wine lover. As a teen, wine was something that my parents sipped and it was either cheap or expensive, white or red, good or bad. I usually quaffed the cheap white stuff (when no one was looking). It was all good to me, and if I drank it cold and fast it could even pass for grape juice with a buzz.

Then in my early twenties, I had the fortunate chance to spend the magical month of May in Paris, and a memorable weekend in Burgundy that, well, changed everything. That spring I memorized only a *soupçon* of the more than 1,000 names and more than 110 appellations in Burgundy, starting, of course, with the Grand Cru vineyards!

I developed a keen taste for what I liked, loved, and could live *sans*. I appreciated the important element of *terrior*–the soil, slope, and environmental conditions–in determining the quality of a burgundy. And I fell in love with the magnificent, elegant, and tricky Pinot Noir grape.

I discovered what is self-evident to every French girl: there's nothing that can't be settled, forgiven, or forgotten over a bottle of wine. "Oh, why Burgundy!" bemoaned my mother, at the news of *mon amour*. A passion for baking, gardening, scrapbooking–or at least New World wines–would have been a preferable (affordable) pursuit for a student.

To this day, wine is one of my greatest passions, deepest loves, and an immeasurable source of pleasure and leisure. Life looks brighter through rosé clinked glasses. *Salut!*

Naughty Tip

On hot days, enjoy *une piscine* (which translates to "swimming pool"): a glass of rosé (or champagne) with ice cubes. Close your eyes and imagine you're sitting poolside in the South of France. As the ice cubes melt, you'll get the added naughty bonus of hydrating while you drink.

When researchers began comparing health in America to health in France several years ago they stumbled upon one of the most well-cited paradoxes in health news: Although the French drink more and consume a significantly higher percentage of dietary fat than Americans, they have significantly lower cholesterol. Scientists ran around frantically trying to figure out *l'ingredient mystère* in the French diet that gave them the healthy edge. They figured it to be one of the active chemical components of red wine: polyphenols. And the media ran wild. *Drink More Wine! Drink to Your Heart's Content!* Still today, the health benefits of vino make headlines.

Resveratrol, a compound found in red grapes, is touted by health media for its antiaging properties. And another ingredient in wine, ellagic acid, has been shown to change the way "fat genes" express themselves, reducing the negative effects they have on weight-loss efforts. Just recently a study came out that found women on a weight-loss program who consumed 10 percent of daily calories from white wine lost about 2 pounds more than did a group that consumed the same number of calories from grape juice.[22]

These studies are all great news. Truly. I'll drink to all of them. Cheers!

But what's not discussed in the clinical journals, or found in polyphenol pills, or resveratrol shots, is the x-factor I discovered in St. Tropez: the relax factor.

The wine-loving French drink and eat in a state of maximum relaxation—at their leisure and in a context of pure pleasure. It's not just the polyphenols that keeps their cholesterol in check, or the resveratrol that keeps them young. It's their parasympathetic nervous system. It's the generous amount of time they take to make (from scratch), enjoy, and celebrate their meals—especially wine.

Alcohol is often one of the first things to go on an old-school, old-rule diet. It's high calorie, high sugar, makes you eat more, and instantly turns into fat, they say. Well, I say they're wrong. And so do top medical minds. While studies suggest alcohol does temporarily inhibit the breakdown of fat cells (your body shifts its metabolic priority to breaking down the alcohol), alcohol alone cannot cause fat storage. Clinical trials also show alcohol actually decreases the appetite over time. In other words, wine doesn't make you fat, it's all the crap you eat with it. I'd much rather you come home from a long day, plunk yourself on the couch, and relax with a glass of wine before dinner (*salad and salmon sounds nice*), than watch you nervously munch through a canister of peanuts while deciding what to have for supper (*Oh, eff it! Chips and cookies.*)

OENOTHERAPY, School of medicine that espouses the belief that wine is penicillin for the nerves. Wine also contains many compounds that have been shown to have health benefits in moderation, including the ethanol, or alcohol, itself. Resveratrol, found in the skins and seeds of grapes, may help prevent cancer, viral infections, and heart disease, and provides anti-aging benefits. Some varieties have more than others.

THE NAUGHTY WINE GLOSSARY

Wine is a matter of taste. It's as simple as
do I like this wine or not? That said,
a basic knowledge of wine will help develop
your tastes, deepen your appreciation,
and impress your friends.

TYPES OF WINE

Pinot Grigio

When it comes to Italian cuisine, we all live by the three *p*'s—pizza, pasta, and pinot grigio, the top-selling imported wine in the United States. Actually a mutation of the red grape pinot noir, pinot grigio appears in France under the name pinot gris. (Same grape—two very different wines.) The Italian pinot grigio usually denotes a light, crisp white, while pinot gris sticks closer to its red grape roots, rich and fuller-bodied with pear and spice flavors.

Pair it! With a body that ranges from anemic to Ah-nold, pinot grigio (a.k.a. gris) can pair with light seafood or wild game depending on its style. In most cases, however, you'll be drinking the lighter, more available grigio.

> Best snack: melon with prosciutto
> Best takeout: sushi
> Best dinner party: pasta with fruits de mer
> Best cookout: grilled summer veggies

Sauvignon Blanc

Easily one of the more characterful and explosive of the popular varietal wines, sauvignon blanc has a variety of styles, all of which include intense aromas and acidity that hit your palate like a kiss from a light socket. The flavors range from tart, minerally, and smoky in its home in France's Loire Valley, to tropical with notes of citrus in California (where it's often called fumé blanc), or grassy and herbal in New Zealand, where this single grape makes up 75 percent of all wine exports.

Pair it! If ever there were a wine for vegetarians, it's sauvignon blanc. The crisp, vegetal flavors make this the go-to wine for stump-the-sommelier foods such as asparagus and artichokes.

Best snack: edamame
Best takeout: Middle Eastern
Best dinner party: roast chicken with lemon
Best cookout: raw oysters

Chardonnay

Like milk, bread, and eggs, chardonnay is an American grocery staple–outselling all other varietal wines. Fortunately for us, there is plenty to go around because chardonnay is planted practically everywhere that wine grapes grow. For this reason, it can be a difficult wine to pin down. One minute it's all lean, crisp, and acidic, as in Chablis, then it's plush, tropical, and buttery when grown in warmer climates and aged in oak. Maybe the versatility is why we love chard so dearly.

Pair it! As a full-bodied white, chardonnay is a classic pairing for poultry and seafood. With big body, a creamy texture, and good acidity, chardonnay also plays well with butter and cream sauces.

Best snack: popcorn
Best takeout: fish and chips
Best dinner party: pasta with Alfredo sauce
Best cookout: steamed lobster

Pinot Noir

Having trouble finding an affordable pinot noir? Blame Hollywood! According to economists, the 2004 movie *Sideways* completely reversed the wine's falling price, with the most dramatic increase in $20 to $40 wines. While it has the lightest body and tannins of the classic red grapes, it can possess a haunting variety of flavors: berries, cola, tea, mushroom, even hints of barnyard. As the lead character Miles eloquently observed, there is something magical about pinot noir.

Pair it! If pinot noir were in grade school, the teacher would give it a gold star for "gets along well with others." This light-bodied red is a peacemaker at any dinner table, able to handle meat, poultry, and flavorful fish with ease.

> Best snack: chips with black bean dip
> Best takeout: Chinese
> Best dinner party: roast duck
> Best cookout: grilled salmon steaks

Zinfandel

Zinfandel is as American as Levis and bank bailouts. Like all red wines, it gets its red color from grape juice coming in contact with the skins. In the 1980s, winemakers left the wine on the skins only briefly to create a sweet, pink wine they dubbed white zinfandel, although it is made from the same red grapes. Now it's white zinfandel, rather than the red stuff, that leads the way in consumption. But whether you like it white and sweet, or red and peppery, zin is worth exploring.

Pair it! With its obvious sweetness, white zinfandel goes well with spicy foods, while the red stuff, with its big berry flavors and medium tannins, is great with tomato dishes and comfort foods like Thanksgiving turkey.

> Best snack: BBQ potato chips
> Best takeout: Mexican
> Best dinner party: eggplant parm
> Best cookout: burgers

Syrah

Syrah is a grape with two different identities, the stately syrah of France's Rhône region and the sassy Australian stuff that prefers to go by shiraz. The best of French syrah (often labeled Côte-Rôtie, Hermitage, or Côtes du Rhône) can be dark and intense, with mineral, pepper, bacon, leather, and tobacco flavors. In a word: rustic. The shiraz of Australia and South Africa tend to be ripe and friendly with blueberry and hints of pepper. In the United States, syrah does well in California and Washington.

Pair it! As a serious red wine, syrah likes serious red meat. The smoky and gamey flavors found in French syrah make it a favorite with lamb, grilled meats, and stews.

Best snack: beef jerky—I adore biltong, from my native South Africa.
Best takeout: gyro
Best dinner party: rack of lamb
Best cookout: grilled sausages

Merlot

It's tough to love cabernet and not love merlot, too. As brothers from Bordeaux, merlot's softer plum, cherry, and coffee flavors are used to balance the more rigid cabernet in classic Bordeaux blends. In California, these blends sometimes go by the name Meritage. Still not convinced? You've probably enjoyed a cab-merlot blend without even realizing it. Often a little cabernet finds its way into a wine labeled merlot and vice versa, as a way to add balance and complexity.

Pair it! With its red fruit and black fruit, full-bodied merlot can handle grilled red meat, while lighter versions are a good choice with poultry or even pasta. The mocha and earthy flavors also work well with mushrooms.

Best snack: dark chocolate
Best takeout: fried chicken
Best dinner party: spaghetti and meatballs
Best cookout: grilled portobello caps

Cabernet Sauvignon

Cabernet is like the high-school quarterback of red grapes: muscular, charismatic, and incredibly popular. Whether bottled alone or in a blend, cabernet brings complexity and power. Its abundance of tannins and generous mouthfeel make this a wine that can handle the heartiest foods. And the best cabs are built to last. With inky dark fruit, such as black cherry and cassis, as well as spicy and herbal flavors of mint and eucalyptus, this grape knows how to wow a crowd.

Pair it! A simple rule is the bigger the wine, the bigger the food. Add to that cabernet's generous tannins, which help to balance food by bonding with fat and protein, and you have the perfect partner for your boldest flavors.

Best snack: empanadas
Best takeout: Philly cheesesteak
Best dinner party: filet mignon
Best cookout: flank or skirt steak

Sparkling Wine

While many Americans are content to fill their day with fizzy cola, for some reason we think sparkling wine is only for wedding toasts and launching ships. While true Champagne, which comes only from the Champagne region of France, can be quite costly, plenty of affordable alternatives from Spain, Italy, Australia, and the United States mean anyone can enjoy a little fizz in their wine. Plus the bubbles and acidity make them some of the most food-friendly and versatile wines around.

Pair it! The bubbling action of sparkling wine, combined with bright acidity, make it like a Roomba for your tongue, ready to clean up after fatty, creamy, salty, or lightly spicy foods.

Best snack: potato chips
Best takeout: French fries
Best dinner party: Parmesan risotto
Best cookout: clambake

HOW TO TALK ABOUT WINE

Aroma All that glass swirling and sniffing isn't just for show. The flavor of a wine, as with other foods, is the result of your taste and smell combined, making aroma an important part of the experience. Some wine grapes are only lightly aromatic, while a few, like Viognier, can smell like imposter perfume. It's all about preference.

Body Think of body as weighing the wine on your tongue. Water is light bodied; cream is heavy bodied; the various milk iterations fall somewhere in between. When matching wine to food, choosing a wine with a similar weight, or body, is usually the best place to start.

Tannin Tannin is found primarily in red wines because they have prolonged contact with grape skins and seeds, where tannins are found naturally. You can sense tannins on your palate as a dry, sometimes gritty, sensation similar to drinking black tea.

Dry *Dry* simply means a wine is without detectable sweetness. Dry wines have less than 2 grams of sugar per liter in them (referred to as residual sugar) and many dry reds have less than 1 gram. However, a demi-sec champagne may have as much as 50 grams per liter. A wine with a hint of sweetness can be called off-dry.

10 QUICK-HIT WAYS TO DECOMPRESS

I know it sounds like an oxymoron: *Quick! Relax!* But desperate times call for naughty measures. When there's no time for a hot bath, it's too early for a glass of wine, and too late for a nap, consider these insta-soothers:

1. Digi-tox. Turn off your phone and ignore your e-mail for 24 hours.
2. Buy some fresh flowers and arrange a bouquet. For you, darling.
3. Lose yourself in a book of poetry.
4. Whistle. You feel pretty sexy and carefree with your lips puckered, don't you? Hold onto that feeling.
5. Listen to the song "Weightless" by Marconi Union. According to the British Academy of Sound Therapy, it is the most relaxing song ever recorded.
6. Brew a pot of herbal tea. That's a pot, not a tea bag. You're not in a rush!
7. Yawn. Release a tunnel of pent-up energy and send a blast of vitamin O to the brain.
8. Sit in a dark room and light one candle. Just one. (Preferably a crystal taper.)
9. Wiggle your toes. Poor man's reflexology.
10. Dig into your naughty drawer and practice self-love . . .

P.S. It's never too early for a glass of wine.

Vintage Simply, the year the grapes were grown for a wine is called its vintage, which is usually expressed by a date on the label. Because grapes are affected by weather, some years are better than others, resulting in good and poor vintages.

Finish This is what's left after you swallow the wine, including the types of flavors and how long they last in your mouth.

And here are fifteen more amazing ideas from the Naughty Survey—they transported me just reading them. Thanks, ladies!

Read on a porch swing

Lie down and listen to a book

Walk 3 miles a day with my dogs

Take a walk—just me and my son

Have a beer and watch a movie with my husband

Horse riding

Capoeira

Playing with the dog

Yoga

Cuddle

Play piano

Admire photos of decorated houses

Smoke weed

Swim

Clean

Masturbate!

CHANGE YOUR BRAIN, CHANGE YOUR BODY

OLD RULE:
Exercise your willpower.

NAUGHTY WAY:
Exercise your imagination.

I KNOW A LOT OF MEN who know a lot about muscles. Should I, for some reason I can't imagine, have a pressing question about beefing up my glutes or shredding my abs or, God forbid, pumping my pecs, there's no shortage of handsome hunks on hand to dispense some workout wisdom.

Now, I love a muscular male physique as much as any girl. My interior psychosexual wallpaper is a manscape of masculine iconography. But whenever my guy friends talk about how big muscles burn the most calories, or insist that deadlifting twice my weight should be a life goal if I really want to get "ripped," I can't help but point out to them that my most efficient fat-burning muscle is just as big as theirs. Maybe bigger.

About one out of every five calories your body burns is smoked not by your glorious glutes or thoroughbred thighs, but by your brain: that sloshy bit of gray gelatin that sits between your diamond studs, directing the whole operation. It may not be constantly pumping like your heart or lungs, or propelling you through the world like your arms and legs, but your brain knows what's up. And your brain–your calorie-burning machine, as big as Tom Brady's, as powerful as LeBron's–is as responsive to proper training as any elite athlete.

Simply put, a lean person has a lean person's brain. This chapter will explain how to get one.

Does This Attitude Make Me Look Fat?

REMEMBER MY YAHOO! PIECE about slim-shaming? The one that got a barrage of brill comments?

But the most thought-provoking e-mail I received was all of two sentences, thirteen words, and two very apropos exclamation points:

Aha! All I had to do was change what was on my fridge!
–Pam

I was trying to be as diligent as I could, responding to everyone who wrote to me, so I didn't read what Pam had written all that closely. I just shot her back what I thought was a clever note:

Dear Pam,
Nothing like a good fridge clear-out to inspire quality
food choices. Hope there's a naughty bottle of champagne
(or two) in there now!   **–M**

Pam wrote back almost instantly.

Not IN the fridge. ON the fridge. I didn't change the contents. Just the magnet!

She went on to tell me her story. She had read a magazine article about a nutritionist who inspired his celebrity clientele by having them post pictures of cows, circus fat ladies, or other cartoonishly rotund characters on their refrigerator–the idea being that once you're reminded of the negative consequences of eating, you'll reject the siren song of the sweets and opt for healthier foods instead.

Until recently she had kept a picture of a pig pinned to the refrigerator. (And on the dashboard of her car.) Each time she approached the kitchen, or the drive-through, she'd be reminded of the consequences of making bad food choices.

But despite what she'd read in the magazine, the strategy backfired; the more Pam looked at that pig, the more piglike she felt. The little sow pinned to her GE fridge was draining all the joy from her food. And if you can't derive pleasure from food–if you're permanently stuck searching for your P-Spot–then it's hard to believe that you deserve quality food. That pig wasn't her ally. It was Food Guilt with a snout!

Inspired by my story of watching the fit and fabulous on the shores of St. Tropez, Pam decided to replace her barnyard pinup with a photo of her favorite beach in Santorini–the beach where she enjoyed her two-week honeymoon. Where she wined and dined on the freshest feta, the sweetest baklava, piles of pita, and lashings of olive oil. Where the only sweat she broke was in bed, and her longest run was the handheld dash she and her husband took from the towel to the sea (and then back to the bedroom). A photo from a time where she felt her most relaxed and adored. Happy, healthy, and sexy as ever.

And I've lost 2 pounds in one week!
Greek goddesses don't do fast, cheap, or easy.
And they don't like Big Macs! Talk about an Aha moment:
Weight loss is just a mind game.

I sent Pam a quick note back:

Dear Greek Goddess Pam. Bingo!
You aren't what you eat.
You are what you think!

Change Your Brain, Change Your Body

WHEN IT COMES TO FOOD, your mind has a mind of its own.

In one study, healthy-weight women who perceived themselves as fat were twice as likely to actually become fat as women who had a more positive, more accurate body image. Talk about a self-fulfilling prophecy!

I also happened upon another study that, while not weight-related, says a lot about our brain's ability to alter our physical appearance. Researchers testing a new chemotherapy treatment found 31 percent of cancer patients who received the placebo–a salt water injection–started losing their hair in exactly the same way a chemo patient would. The only reason for the side effect? The patients believed their hair loss was an inevitability.

If the mind is powerful enough to make our hair fall out when ingesting salt water, what do you think happens when we tell ourselves: "This burger is going straight to my thighs"?

But as the command center from which every Naughty thought and instinct arises, your brain is as eager to learn as a new puppy, even if you've been feeding it nothing more taxing than a steady diet of *Scandal*. Swedish researchers who looked at the effect of cognitive behavioral therapy (a type of psychotherapy that works to change negative thinking) saw participants lose up to 17 pounds in ten weeks–simply from training the brain to "think like a thin person."[1] Through a series of courses, written tests, and follow-ups, the subjects were taught simple, new ways to think about food–for example, thinking of hunger as normal and tolerable, as opposed to something dramatic that needs to be solved immediately.

MIND GAMES

Your subconscious is a moonscape pockmarked with suppositions—long-ago dents made in the way you feel about yourself, your body, and your relationship with food. If you want to change the way your subconscious thinks about food, you need to throw your consciousness a curveball. The following seven exercises are inspired by Japanese *kaon*, mental puzzles designed to help Zen students let go of their basic assumptions about the rational world. But much naughtier, of course. . . .

1. Learn how to order your favorite meal, cocktail, and coffee in another language.

2. Eat with your nondominant hand.

3. Order dessert before your main course. Finish with an appetizer.

4. Light a birthday candle and make a wish on any day other than your birthday.

5. Try a food you have never eaten, like escargots.

6. Slip on very sexy lingerie before running very ordinary errands.

7. Make a reservation under a pseudonym and assume the character for the duration of the meal. *Breakfast for two? Right this way, Miss Golightly . . .*

In a way, the whole Naughty Diet is a big cognitive behavioral guidebook. Together, you and I are going through the process of changing the way we think about food. But CBT, as it's known in the field, is a drawn-out process that really needs an expert to guide you. In the course of my research, I've stumbled upon a shortcut. A very Naughty one.

You Are Getting Sleepy . . . Very Sleepy . . .

LET ME TELL YOU about my two most favorite moments of the day. One happens first thing in the morning, that hazy moment when I'm just waking up and the alarm hasn't yet slapped me in the face with its cold, fishy palm. It's that narcotic, dreamlike state where fantasy and reality meet. A glimmer of light is starting to weave through my eyelids; there's a warm body next to me. Am I still at that world premiere with a Hemsworth brother on each arm? Pieces of my reality slowly gather to form a picture like those metal shavings drawn with a magnetic pencil. My dreams are right there, in my grasp, but slipping away by the second.

My other favorite moment? It comes at the end of the evening, when the process happens in reverse–often accelerated by a glorious romp, endorphins firing away and then simmering down into cozy embers. And what makes these moments so gloriously peaceful?

Hypnosis.

That's what I learned from a long talk with Nazanin Barlavi, a therapist who has her own practice, Hypnotherapy Wellness, in California. "That feeling that you're not completely awake but you're not asleep either? It means you're in hypnosis, or a meditative state," she says. "What that means is that your brain waves are in an alpha state. You become very suggestible to your environment. You're not entirely conscious, and your subconscious mind is profoundly more powerful."

Your subconscious mind, says Nazanin, makes up about 88 percent of your total brain power. That's where all your memories, associations, and–most important–habits and identity are stored. "It's kind of like a hard drive," she says. "A hard drive that's been building ever since you were born."

And that's the reason it's so hard to change our instinct to be "good" or "worthy" or our habits of reaching for something nasty when we feel bad. "Once an unhelpful thought gets stored in that hard drive–that a whole pizza offers comfort, or that carbs are inherently bad–it's very hard to shake without getting into that hard-drive and deleting the file."

And the master programmer of that hard drive, says Nazanin, is Guilt. "A lot of my clients who struggle with weight and food issues also feel a sense

YEAH, BABY!

Chances are, if you're coming from old-school, old-rule diet territory, you're pretty well versed in telling your mind no. But the subconscious doesn't hear negatives. Tell yourself often enough that you will never eat carbs, you shouldn't eat sweets, you don't do dessert on weeknights, and you will not eat a slice of cake, and you've charted a course toward a very big binge.

Every chance you get to embrace an opportunity by saying yes is a special occasion—a moment of acceptance, gratitude, healthy control, and pleasure. Practice replacing the dark, guilty cloud of NO with the expansive sky of YES!

- Certainly!
- My thoughts exactly.
- Is the pope Catholic?
- I'd love that!
- Book it, Dano!
- *Mais oui!*
- Believe you me.
- *Ja.*
- Aye, my lady.
- No diggity.
- You bet your boots!
- Let's!
- Sold!
- Why not?

of guilt in their lives, and they've formed a subconscious belief somewhere along the way that they need to emotionally protect themselves with their weight, or that eating provides a coping mechanism when they feel anxious or guilty."

Since many people eat from their subconscious—almost automatically—tapping into that hard drive and training the mind to think differently can be profoundly effective. "People think they can solve these food issues with willpower, on a conscious level, and they don't understand why they keep going back," Nazanin says. "What's ironic is that so many people seek out psychotherapists to help with weight loss, and that is solely cognitive–conscious–therapy. The problem is not your conscious mind; it's your subconscious."

Is it effective? There's one hypnotherapist in England who is in high demand for his "virtual gastric band surgery"; instead of opting for the real thing–a drastic surgery for weight loss in which a silicone strap is clamped around the stomach, reducing the amount of food a person can eat–his patients are persuaded, under hypnosis, that they've actually had the operation and are physically incapable of eating a big meal.

But that doesn't sound particularly Naughty. Our goal isn't to render ourselves incapable of indulgence. It's to enjoy the food, skip the guilt, and reap the physical and emotional benefits.

Resetting Your Hard Drive

FOOD ISSUES DON'T come from the mean girls in high school, or the media, or that guy who broke it off with you on your twenty-first birthday. They started long before that.

"Your subconscious is constantly communicating with you and storing files on that hard drive," Nazanin says. "But when you were born, from zero to eight years old, you were most suggestible. Whatever your family or friends told you between those ages, whether it was true or not, you believed it. If someone told you that you were fat, or if you grew up with a mother who berated her own body or was constantly dieting–that affected you deeply. Hypnotherapy is a matter of tapping into the subconscious and creating new belief systems and changing those associations."

Nazanin then walked me through a series of self-hypnosis techniques which, in the interest of all that is Naughty, I began practicing on myself. And honestly, it was not easy–at first. "If you're a left-brain, serious, logical person who is always in her head, it can take a little time to warm up to hypnosis," Nazanin explained. But, she assured me, we are all our own best hypnotherapist. "You're actually most suggestible to your own suggestions because you believe and trust yourself the most."

Here's how to play the ultimate mind game on yourself:

- Make sure that you're well fed, well hydrated, and totally comfortable. Get into some cozy clothes.

- Set yourself up in a recliner, or on your bed with some pillows propping yourself up. You're going to want to dance along the edge of sleep, but not fall into it.

- Put a blanket over yourself. A blanket provides a sense of security, comfort, and warmth, exactly what you need to get into a fully relaxed state.

- Find a spot on the wall or ceiling and, with your eyes open, focus all of your attention on that spot. After a few minutes, you'll start noticing that your breathing is getting a little heavier. Your eyes may start blinking, and you may feel the need to swallow. This means you're beginning to fall into a state of deep relaxation.

- Now, close your eyes. Take three deep breaths into your belly. Open your mind. You're ready to begin.

Imagine a beautiful bright golden sphere is hovering over your head. It's absorbing all the anxiety, the Guilt, the worry. Visualize this sphere traveling through your body, absorbing the tension–starting at your head, down to your throat, your neck, your shoulders, your spine–all the way down to your toes.

Now, visualize yourself standing at the top of a staircase. You're walking down twenty steps. And with each step, you're feeling more and more relaxed.

You're at the bottom of the steps now. Say to yourself–in your head, or out loud–"Deep sleep."

You're now looking at three doors: a golden door, a green door, and a purple door. Pick your favorite door. Turn the knob, and go to the other side.

You find yourself in a very relaxing place–a garden, a forest; it could even be Mojito Beach. Activate all of your senses: Smell the fresh air. Hear the winds whisper or the waves crashing. Feel the sunshine on your body.

As you start to walk along the beach, visualize the weight shedding with every step: The pounds, the Guilt, the pressure. Every step, you're getting closer to your goal.

Imagine yourself feeling healthy. You're wearing that little black dress, or those tight jeans you've always wanted to fit into to. You look beautiful. You are beautiful.

Now is the moment when you'll want to start feeding your subconscious suggestions, as if they have already happened. So, you want to say things in your head, like: *I am healthy. I am confident. I am motivated. I am gorgeous and vibrant.* You're reprogramming your subconscious mind–which may have been taught different lessons about who you are.

Once you're ready to leave your little dreamland, find the door that led you there. Turn the knob, climb the staircase. As you reach the top, start counting yourself back into consciousness: "One, two, three, four, five. Eyes open, wide awake."

Self-hypnosis is a process that takes some practice to get right. Naza-

THE NAUGHTY ROLE MODELS

Whether you're heading out for a night on the town, or fixing yourself a bowl of oatmeal, it's helpful to have a handful of naughty characters in mind to inspire your every move.* Everyone has her own idea of healthy-sexy. Identify a few women who inspire *you* to live a naughtier lifestyle, or peruse this list:

AUDREY HEPBURN, for being Audrey

EVE, for being a confident, badass babe who proved men are ignorant until women feed them

TAYLOR SWIFT, for making Apple back down with one mighty Tweet

ADELE, for owning her body, and not letting it be owned

MINDY KALING, for saying what we're all thinking

MARIE ANTOINETTE, for letting us eat cake

nin recommends trying it at least twice a week in the evenings, for about twenty minutes at a time. But if this idea seems just too foreign to you, there are some cheats you can try to get your subconscious in shape. Here are the techniques that worked for me:

The dream board. As part of the process of creating this book, I began to put together a "mood board." But as I immersed myself more and more in the images I created, I discovered a sort of natural calm and focus coming over me. The more images I collected, the more I began to relate to those images. "Make a vision board," says Nazanin. "Make it bold and big and beautiful, because that's how your subconscious mind works—through images. Put it up on your wall and look at it every day. Before you know it, all those things are going to start appearing in

CHARLIZE THERON, for being a South African legend, a supermodel beauty, family homicide survivor, Oscar winner, badass, etc. etc. . . .

ANGELA MERKEL, **CHRISTINE LAGARDE**, and **JANET YELLEN**, for being the three most powerful economic decision-makers in the world

JULIA CHILD, for reminding us that butter and cream are nothing to fear

VICTORIA BECKHAM, for showing that even the world's sexiest man can find one woman enough

CLEOPATRA, for being a supreme seductress

EMMELINE PANKHURST, for embodying the naughty expression "Well-behaved women rarely make history."

* You can certainly be more than one woman at once.
As in gemstones, facets add sparkle and intrigue to every brilliantly complex Naughty Girl.

your life. Your subconscious mind will be working for you. It's all about learning how to make your subconscious mind work for you, and not the other way round."

Think back to Pam, and her images of the pig on the refrigerator. Subconsciously, she was suggesting to herself that she was, in fact, pig-like. Overcoming food guilt was impossible when she found herself staring at it day after day.

The dream meal. This one was fun. Each morning, as I woke up, I'd think about foods that I wanted that day–there's an incredible Italian place a few blocks away with a tiramisu that can bring tears to your eyes. I fantasized about a huge wedge, creamy mocha-flavored dream. Later that week, a girlfriend and I shared a piece over gossip and espressos. And my food fantasy helped make portion control automatic.

Research shows that imagining yourself eating a certain food may help you consume less of it when you actually indulge. It's exactly why discipline and self-denial don't work. Instead of trying to tamp down your cravings, indulge them. Enjoy them openly. Fantasize about them. A little bit of decadence in your dendrites helps make real-world discipline much easier.

The dream dress. A year ago, I had splurged on a long, white silk Givenchy gown. The couture cut was so exquisite it enveloped my body like a delicate second skin. But over the winter when an extended bout of stress hit, I took a simultaneous hiatus from both my gym membership and my common sense in the kitchen. The resulting pooch–barely noticeable in my every day clothes–rendered the silk sheath a catastrophe. The feminine lines suddenly bunched at my waist and made me feel like that poor blueberry-shaped girl from *Charlie and the Chocolate Factory.*

I took a page from Nazanin's book, and imagined myself back in that slip of a dress–slim, sexy, and at my peak physical condition. I imagined myself fresh from a workout, my torso tight and toned. And, at her suggestion, I hung the dress on the door of my closet, where I'd see it every day as I emerged from sleep. "Since your subconscious works in images, seeing that dress will trigger those same thin, beautiful, sexy, confident feelings," Nazanin told me. I told myself the story of getting back to the gym, eating healthier, and fitting into the Givenchy. My subconscious learned the story too—and that's how it became a reality.

Those women who stay "naturally thin," who seem to have it all together without dieting, without sacrificing, without re-creating the Bataan Death March on their treadmill each morning? You can't ask them their secret, because they don't have one. Or rather, they don't know that they have one, because their secret is a secret even from them. It's buried deep in their subconscious, a naughty fairy godmother implanted in early childhood who watches out for them at every turn.

And now you know the secret of conjuring one up for yourself . . . !

A Word on Exercise
Chase Your Joy

WHEN I WAS A CHILD, I don't think I even knew the meaning of *exercise*.

Oh, I got plenty of it. I was a master tree climber, an obsessive swimmer, a neighborhood champion in the universal sport of freeze tag. The sight of a playground set could send my whole body into a frenzy of energy that I couldn't wait to burn off.

Then, somewhere around age twelve, I discovered my boobs and boys. And soon after, exercise entered my world as a nasty chore.

MTV had just come to South African cable, and music videos sporting beautiful bodies motivated me to start running and do one hundred daily crunches for Kevin Huxom, my teenage crush. Shortly after, my mom purchased a medieval torture device known as the Health Walker, which required the user to swing her legs back and forth in a sort of straight-legged goosewalk. She wisely never used it, so I moved it into my room.

I positioned the dreaded device on one side of my room, while on the opposite wall I hung a poster from *Titanic* ("You're the king of my world, Leo!"), a photo of Esther Cañades that I'd torn from the pages of *Vogue*, and, in my own handwriting, the words DON'T EAT! JUST SWING! Every day for two hours I'd rock myself back and forth until the rudimentary pedometer on it registered ten thousand swings, enough to earn myself Esther's body and Leo's love. A DO NOT DISTURB sign hung on my bedroom door kept my parents at bay–and no doubt had them convinced they were raising a hermit.

When I grew up and moved to London, running became my obsession. Regardless of how I felt, physically or emotionally, I pushed my body to run at least 8 miles every other day. I pounded out the miles on a treadmill, staring blankly at the cracked beige wall of the Virgin Active, not wanting to be distracted by the TV sets that floated overhead. On days when the bitter British rains receded, I'd take to the streets, looping through the parks and dreaming of all the food I'd earned through my ritual of self-punishment. Sure, I enjoyed a few bouts of "runner's high"–or at least the "I'm on the home stretch" high and "I can eat guilt-free tonight" high. But what I'd become was runorexic–my entire self-worth could be measured in miles and calories.

Imagine then what happened when the very thing I built that self-worth on began to crumble.

It started with a bit of an ache at the front of my lower leg that would set in after a run. Of course, I ignored it. And of course, it continued to deepen.

Soon, each footfall felt like a baseball bat to my shins. When I could stand it no longer, I hobbled into a chiropractor.

"Shin splints," he explained. "Pretty severe. You need to rest."

I remember tears welling up silently. I pursed my mouth to keep my lower lip from trembling. *What will I eat? I thought. How will I eat? What if I still want to eat like a runner? What if . . . I get fat?*

RUNOREXIC, One who runs obsessively to control and maintain their weight. Usually found on the same treadmill at the gym, with an Exorcist-level over-focus.

Born to run

I STILL RUN, but today I run very differently.

I used to run away from things: I ran away from my feelings, away from my fear, away from my hunger and insecurity. I *couldn't* stop running, no matter how much pain I felt, because if I did, those dark shadows might catch up to me.

Now I run to catch things. I run to catch joy, pleasure, energy, and freedom. I run to catch a buzz. I run to play out my fantasies. Sometimes when I run, I'm Lara Croft, kicking zombie ass. Sometimes I'm just me, Melissa, and that boy on the bike who just whizzed by is Leo D.–I've got to catch him! ("Remember me? The girl from the Health Walker?") And sometimes I'm eight-year-old me, running without ego or any higher purpose than to burn off extra energy and feel the wind in my hair.

When I'm Lara Croft, one more mile seems easy breezy. Burpees? How many?! When I'm chasing something I want, kicking it into the next gear comes effortlessly. When I run without fear or ego, I'm not at work, I'm at play. I don't always time myself on my runs, but when I do, it's because I'm enjoying the competition; I want today me to be a little faster, a little fitter than yesterday me. And if it's too cold to run outside, then I'm taking the day off. (Sorry/not sorry: I have self-diagnosed PTSD: post-treadmill stress disorder.)

Chasing joy works for me. (Hey, I can still fit into my high school uniform for Halloween.) But how can I prescribe my fitness routine for you? As with diet, trying to force you to do my workout makes no sense. Maybe you hate running. Maybe you have an allergy to polycarbonate soles. Maybe you live in a frozen wasteland covered with ice. I don't know. But I do know that trying to force you to do my workout is going to lead us right back to where we started.

To solve this exercise enigma, I got on the phone with Ariane Smith Machin, PhD, a licensed clinical and sport psychologist who works with athletes and others who want to improve their body and their mind. And she confirmed what I'd intuited on my own.

"Letting joy dictate how and when you exercise is *exactly* what will bring longevity to your fitness routine," she explained. "When you focus your goals on *feeling good*, the aesthetic goals–looking killer in that dress or bikini–just come naturally.

"Everyone has a different idea of what type of fitness will bring them joy," Ariane continued. "You decide what activity works for you, what makes you happy, what you can afford; and you move forward from there. Be forgiving in the process."

So, it's okay if I . . . ummmm . . . skipped my planned run today and danced around in my new Agent Provocateur set for 40 minutes instead? I wondered.

"You've gotta forget the rules and the shoulds. Let all that go. Do some thinking about the kind of movement that brings you pleasure and joy. Don't compare yourself to anyone else. It doesn't have to be a 5k, though it could be. It doesn't have to include weights, though it could. It could just be the joy of taking your dog for a walk, playing with your kids, or dancing around your room in your lingerie."

Huzzah!

Then she threw me some questions of her own: "Did you move for twenty minutes today, M?"

"Yes! At least!" I said.

"And did it bring you joy?"

"Lots!"

"Did you feed your body properly–not restrict and not overeat?"

"Yep," I said, eyeing the gorgeous fresh baguette I was planning to slather with Brie as soon as our call ended.

"Well, bravo! Fist bump! You're ahead of a lot of people."

Simply hearing Dr. Ariane affirm my naughty fitness philosophy boosted my personal stores of joy. I used to feel guilty when I "only did dance workouts"–they were almost too fun to be effective, I thought. That's when I'd start comparing and doubting; and feel that perhaps I should be lifting bars or doing barre like my friend with the hottest ass ever. Or yoga ("It's life-changing," said my yogi friend). Or Pilates. Or . . .

STOP!

Fact is, Naughty Girl, feeling good is fundamental to looking good. If you've already found the types of exercise that feel good to you, keep going. If you need a bit of joy-chasing inspiration, check out my list of 101 Fun & Flirty Ways to Get Moving on naughtydiet.com. It's okay to try something and hate it, just don't give up. Find a handful of things that bring you joy: a few low-intensity exercises for weight maintenance and active rest days and some more intense forms that will get your heart rate up. Aim to move for twenty minutes a day–it doesn't have to be all at once, though it could be.

Keep chasing joy. It's the pursuit, not the end goal, which matters most.

Vanity Flair

IF YOU'RE AN AVOWED exercise-phobe who can't imagine taking the next step toward fitness, then here's what I want you to do. Take that old baggy tee-shirt you wore the last time you worked out. Yea, that one. And that one. And the sweatpants, too. Take a pair of scissors and cut them into squares. They're no longer your workout clothes. But, hey! You now have rags to clean the house.

Research shows people describe themselves in a way that's consistent with how they dress. That's why it's a terrible idea to save old, ratty clothes as "workout clothes." If you don't feel good when you work out, then you're not going to work out. And a huge part of feeling good is looking good. Dr. Ariane calls it "dress-ercize." You don't need to spend a lot of money, or dress in head-to-toe spandex–though if that's what makes you feel best, by all means!

The key is finding clothes that you feel comfortable in. That could be all black, neon, print–whatever works. (Just stay away from gray leggings! Nothing is more horrifying and demotivating than crack sweat.)

A few more dos and don'ts:

DO invest in a few proper-fitting sports bras. If you're small-chested, you'll probably feel best in something padded that doesn't leave you looking flat as a board. And if you're busty (lucky!), invest in something that keeps the girls safely fastened, so you don't have to worry about any undesirable bouncing or sagging.

DON'T wear makeup. It really just looks silly, not to mention it's terrible for your skin. Mascara is fine, unless you're swimming. And please: no perfume or heavily scented body lotions. I'm sure it smells lovely, but fragrance is designed to interact with our body at resting temperature (that's why you test it on "pulse points"). When you get hot, your *eau de toilette* becomes *eau de regret*–very strong, very musky and just . . . nasty.

DO wear the right pair of shoes for the right activity. The right shoes can make you feel lighter, faster, and stronger; the wrong shoes will not only make your workout feel harder, they could cause an injury. It's the one bit of exercise equipment every person should invest in.

DON'T force yourself to perform exercises that are painful, awkward, or make you feel stupid. There are dozens of ways to work every muscle in your body; don't do the ones that make you feel ridiculous. (One of those fitness-obsessed boys I mentioned earlier admits that he won't do certain exercises because they don't make him feel cool. "I won't lunge," he says. "I don't care if it's the best overall leg exercise, it looks goofy. On the other hand, I have a very strong back. Because pull-ups always look cool.")

Naughty Activity
PAMPER YOURSELF

Rewarding yourself for your efforts with a self-care ritual is a great way to motivate yourself. Maybe you'll treat yourself to a massage or a manicure, buy a new lippie, or hem your favorite dress an inch shorter to show off your new gorgeous gams. A little pampering can go a long way towards boosting your body confidence, and it prevents you from rewarding your workout with takeout. Remember: Self-care is not selfish! When you take steps to take care of your body, you'll feel more beautiful, more confident, and more able to share yourself with others.

Naughty Quiz
What's Your Naughty Fitness Personality?

You wouldn't buy a dress that didn't "feel right," and you wouldn't commit to a man who left you feeling *blah*. Choosing the right exercise routine is no different. Finding a workout that suits your fitness personality means you'll be more likely to stick with it long term. If you love your current workout, then rock on. But if you're looking for something new, take this simple self-test:

1. The best workouts are:

(a) Hard

(b) Quick

(c) Fun

2. You're just about to head to the gym when your phone rings. It's your bestie cross-country whom you rarely hear from. You:

(a) Decline call. You'll call back after the gym.

(b) Speed walk and talk for hours. You love sneaking in the exercise.

(c) Dump your bag, sit on the couch and gab. Girls before curls.

3. When you see a workout plan in a magazine, you usually:

(a) Study it for ideas and tips on form.

(b) Tear it out with good intentions to try but never actually do it.

(c) Remark at how thin the model is then flip the page without reading it.

4. You prefer to exercise:

   (a) At the same time every day, barring unforeseen circumstances.

   (b) Whenever you feel inspired!

   (c) When your friends will join you.

5. A piece of IKEA furniture arrives in five boxes. The first thing you do is:

   (a) Read the instruction manual. Twice.

   (b) Pour a glass of wine, and have at it. Sans instructions. You like a challenge!

   (c) Call your sweetie for help.

6. When it comes to fitness advice for a healthy-sexy body, you're more likely to trust:

   (a) Peer-reviewed studies and evidence-backed papers.

   (b) Gisele's trainer.

   (c) The girls in the front row at your favorite group-exercise class.

7. The best preworkout is:

   (a) Black coffee or green tea.

   (b) A glass of wine. Or an invite for a glass of wine somewhere fancy.

   (c) A pep talk.

8. The fitness gadget you're most likely to have is:

   (a) A heart rate monitor

   (b) A Fitbit

   (c) Sneakers. They count, right?

9. Do you have to sweat to feel like you've had a good workout?

(a) Not necessarily.

(b) No; you actually prefer workouts that leave you looking fresh and dewy.

(c) Yes. Sweat is my fat crying.

10. The mantra that motivates you most is:

(a) No pain, no gain.

(b) Good enough is good enough.

(c) Just do it.

11. You eat a cupcake on a day you planned to go to the gym. How does this affect your workout?

(a) You punish yourself for the unplanned indulgence with an extra hour of cardio.

(b) The sugar gives you a rush of energy that makes the workout whiz by.

(c) You skip the gym. You've already blown it.

12. The kind of workout instructor who motivates you most is:

(a) You!

(b) Your fantasies of Leo DiCaprio.

(c) The peppy one with the killer playlist.

13. Your favorite rest-day activity is:

(a) Hot yoga and a long hike in the woods.

(b) A long walk and a longer nap.

(c) Hanging out with friends.

14. You see a segment on the news about a new fitness trend that includes hula hooping. You think:

    (a) Eye roll. Fads are a waste of time.

    (b) I have a hula hoop! I should try that at home.

    (c) Must text friends immediately and try to find a class.

15. The special man in your life suggests you go for a run together. You think:

    (a) Fun! Hope I can keep up . . .

    (b) Can't we do some bedroom cardio instead?

    (c) He must think I'm fat.

16. When you're on vacation, you . . .

    (a) Try to stick to your regular workout schedule to compensate for the extra food and alcohol.

    (b) Take a break from "traditional" exercise, and figure that swimming in the sea, walking along the beach and having sex is enough to stay healthy.

    (c) Hardly move! But you might try a beach yoga class.

17. Your personal trainer is a no-show for your sixty-minute session. You:

    (a) Do the same workout solo.

    (b) HIIT it for 20 minutes and quit it.

    (c) Go home and pout.

18. The hardest part about your fitness routine is:

    (a) Making it challenging enough.

    (b) Trying not to get bored.

    (c) Getting started.

19. You see a healthy-sexy woman at the gym doing a hard-core CrossFit-style workout. You think:

(a) Her form could be better.

(b) She's so hot! Maybe I should be doing that . . .

(c) Ugh, I'm so fat. I'll never look like that.

20. When it comes to fitness attire you prioritize:

(a) What makes my workout most effective

(b) What makes me feel sexy and confident

(c) What makes me feel comfortable

21. It's pouring rain and you had planned to go for a run. You:

(a) Change into a black tank top and go anyway.

(b) Do some yoga in your living room instead.

(c) Skip working out today.

22. The best free weights to use are:

(a) Heavier than last time.

(b) Household objects like groceries and wine bottles.

(c) Pink.

23. You go out to dinner at your favorite restaurant after a killer workout earlier that day. This means:

(a) You're inspired to make healthy choices so as not to "erase" your hard work.

(b) You can enjoy your favorite dish, guilt free!

(c) You can reward yourself with a decadent dessert.

Naughty Quiz: **Scorecard**

Mostly a's:
THE FITNESS FANATIC

As someone who identifies as a planner, you take a reserved, routine approach to fitness, sticking to familiar, tried-and-true exercises. You like to have all the facts before making a decision and prefer to go it alone. Your competitive, Type A nature is both a help and a hindrance. Self-discipline comes naturally, but your rigidity and need for control can lead to neurotic tendencies. Your exercise routine could afford some flexibility, rest time, and a little more naughtiness.

Naughty prescription for more joy: Build a few active rest days into your routine every week–go for a walk, take a yoga class, or just get yourself a deep tissue massage. Retrain your brain to consider this peaceful, healing time as much a priority for reaching and maintaining your healthy-sexy goals as the time you're "on." Try a new form of exercise once a week, preferably something fluid like dancing or swimming. Stay away from fitness apps and gadgets that fuel unhealthy neurotic tendencies.

Mostly b's:
THE FITNESS FLIRT

A true naughty spirit, you find traditional forms of working out boring. You prefer dancing in your room to taking a Zumba class, and you're always looking for shortcuts that get you more for less. Your improvisational approach to exercise is to be admired, but your tendency to get bored and chronically compare yourself with others gets in the way of a routine you can stick with long term. You can get turned off to the idea of working out just as soon as you can get turned on. Your fitness routine needs some inspiration and affirmation.

Naughty prescription for more joy: Take a cue from Dr. Ariane, and when you start panicking whether you're "doing enough" or "doing the right thing," ask yourself "Did I move today? Did I nourish myself with naughty, high-quality foods?" Work on affirming your intentions and you'll find yourself moving and grooving more and more. You might also benefit from a Fitbit or app that will keep you motivated to keep moving throughout the day and help you to ease up on old school "sweat for thirty minutes at a time in a gym" mentality.

Mostly c's:
THE FITNESS FOLLOWER

When it comes to fitness, you're all about the social experience. You tend to favor relationships over results, and having fun is most important to you in a workout. You're externally motivated–by the acceptance of others, by rewards, and by trends (and food!)–but you have a hard time giving yourself the same kick in the butt. Your casual exercise routine is in need of a sense of commitment and intrinsic motivation.

Naughty prescription for more joy: Don't fight your social butterfly status: group classes and finding friends who want to work out are both great for you; team sports, CrossFit gyms, and even participating in 5ks (walk if you must!) can offer the same sense of community and challenge. Work on motivating yourself by finding nonfood rewards: schedule a spa day, or slip $1 in a jar every day you work out and buy yourself a sexy new workout outfit with the funds.

18 NAUGHTY TRICKS FOR GETTING MORE OUT OF DOING LESS

Naughty Girls love a good shortcut, especially when it comes to getting the max fat-burn and healthy-sexy muscle tone from a minimal-effort fitness plan. Here are eighteen ways to triple the effectiveness of your workout, and get more out of doing less:

1. **Pregame With Green Tea.** I took a preworkout supplement once and felt like I had swallowed a box of fireworks. Not to mention the insane itch that followed (no thanks, beta alanine). Now I get my caffeine boost with green tea, and get the added benefit of torching more fat from every run. In a recent *study*, participants who combined a daily habit of four or five cups of green tea each day with a 25-minute sweat session lost 2 more pounds than the non-tea-drinking exercisers.[2]

2. **Move Before You Munch.** Breaking a sweat before breakfast could get you into your skinny jeans faster. According to some studies, exercising in a fasted state can burn almost *20 percent more fat* compared to exercising with fuel in the tank.[3] That's because once your glucose stores (the food/carbs in your system) are depleted, your body has to use its own fat for fuel.

3. **HIT It, Then Quit It.** On days when you really can't be arsed, just move for two and a half minutes. Research published in the journal *Physiological Reports* showed that people who did five eighty-second bursts of max-effort exercise burned 200 extra calories that day—not that we're counting.[4] (But if we did, we'd know that extra effort just afforded us two more glasses of vino. Cheers!)

4. **Get Paid.** Stop spending money on trainers who'll keep you accountable and start earning money for your efforts instead. Research found that people who were paid $100 to go to the gym doubled their attendance rate.[5] Don't have a sugar daddy? Check out apps like Pact, in which fellow users will pay you hard cash to stick to your schedule. If

you miss your session, you authorize the app to charge your credit card. When you reach your goal, you get paid out of a common pool.

5. **Avoid the Mirror.** "But I need to check my form!" Yeah, yeah. Chances are, if you're addicted to your own reflection at the gym, you're not checking your form; you're checking your flab. Stop it! You're only stressing yourself out. FACT: One study found that women who exercised in front of a mirror felt less calm and more fatigued after a 30-minute workout than did those who weren't staring at their reflection.[6]

6. **Go "OM" . . .** Run on the treadmill for long enough and you'll enter "the zone"—a mental state psychologists refer to as "flow" that occurs naturally and makes us feel deceptively stronger, fitter, and more focused. But research suggests people who meditate can get in the zone faster. One study found that people's "flow" dispositions increased, and their workouts optimized, with just twenty minutes of meditation practice a day.[7]

7. **Do Laundry Like You Mean It!** When one group of hotel maids was told the movement they did during their day jobs exceeded the surgeon general's guidelines for fitness, they started losing weight, according to a study published in *Association for Psychological Science*.[8] In fact, after a month, the average maid had dropped 2 pounds! Study authors attribute the results to the positive impact of self-awareness and engagement. Approach your daily chores with gusto and verve, Cinderelly, and watch your body transform.

8. **Pretend a Hot Guy is Running Behind You.** 'Nuff said.

9. **Sign a Contract.** You can make promises to yourself that you WILL work out all the livelong day, but research suggests you're more likely to actually follow through if you sign a contract in front of someone.[9] According to study authors, you can make the pledge even more effective if you build in a penalty—agreeing to pay your witness (or a jar) $5 every time you bail, for instance. Participants who signed longer contracts ended up exercising more than those who agreed to shorter ones, so pull out a lippie and sign

a long-term agreement. *I will move my arse for at least ten to twenty minutes every day, so help me, Naughty God!*

10. **Grab a Weight.** Or a bottle of wine. Or a cantaloupe. Or a small child (preferably one you know). Adding just three sessions of "heavy lifting" a week can reduce your body fat by 3 percent, without cutting calories, according to research.[10] Another study in the journal *Medicine & Science in Sports & Exercise* found women who lifted more weight for fewer reps burned nearly twice as many calories than when they did more with a lighter weight.[11] (So, upgrade to a magnum of champs, a watermelon, or a toddler.)

11. **Rock Your Blue Jeans.** Kick off your heels and keep it casual. A study by the American Council on Exercise suggests casual clothing, as opposed to conventional business attire, can increase physical activity levels in our daily routines.[12] Participants in the study took an additional 491 steps, and burned 25 more calories, on days they wore denim than when they wore traditional business clothes. That may sound trivial, but the calories add up: Researchers say keeping it casual just once a week could slash 6,250 calories over the course of the year–enough to offset the average annual weight gain (0.4 to 1.8 pounds) experienced by most Americans.

12. **Run, Rave, Repeat.** Make a naughty don't-sweat-it playlist of your favorite jams. A study in *Journal of Sport & Exercise Psychology* found participants who ran on a treadmill and kept in strict time with the beat of motivational pop music were able to run 15 percent longer than usual and feel more positive–even when working out at a high intensity close to exhaustion.[13]

13. **And Make it "Happy."** If you really want to take your HIIT session to the next level, download the song "Happy" by Pharrell Williams. A sports psychology analysis of more than 6.7 million Spotify playlists found the beats in the song most closely match the stride rate of high-intensity cardio.[14]

14. Stop Loafing. You'll torch 37 percent more calories if you cut rests between sets from three minutes to eighty seconds, a College of New Jersey study found.[15] You'll also get it over with faster. So, you can go to cocktail hour sooner.

15. Motivate with Text Messages. A study published in the *Journal of Nutrition and Behavior* showed that college students who received regular text "nudges" to their smartphone that reminded them to eat better and exercise more engaged in slightly more rigorous physical activity than those who didn't receive the text messages.[16] So, solicit a text buddy to be your get-healthy-sexy coach, or take matters into your own hands; set up labeled alarms on your smartphone.

16. Give Yourself a Pep Talk. Repeat: *I am a toned Naughty goddess! I feel great! I love burpees!* A study in the journal *Medicine & Science in Sports & Exercise* found that cyclists who systematically verbalized positive affirmations (either silently or aloud) were able to pedal for much longer–and also said it felt easier–than their counterparts who skipped the consistent pep talk.[17] Researchers say the data suggests motivational self-talk can dramatically improve endurance performance; and, on a deeper level, a horrible workout may really be in your head!

17. Fend Off a Nasty Postworkout Binge. Naughty weapon: watermelon. Super yummy, super low-cal and mostly water that will help rehydrate your naughty bod, the juicy fruit also has the added benefit of reducing fat accumulation, according to research conducted at the University of Kentucky.[18] Better yet, a study among athletes by the Universidad Politécnica de Cartagena in Spain found watermelon juice to help reduce the level of muscle soreness–so you can get back at it tomorrow.[19]

18. Take a Nap. You need those seven to nine hours of shut-eye to keep you energized throughout the day and during your workout. A recent study found subpar sleep could undermine weight loss by as much as 55 percent! One more reason to linger a little longer, baby.[20]

The Naughty Workout
–for Two

Remember Sharon on Mojito Beach, who was feeling distant from her husband after raiding her mini-fridge for Toblerones? She should have done this workout. All you need is a lover and a towel–that's my idea of the perfect gym equipment! Besides being great for your butt, legs, tris and thighs, this routine, compliments of *The Bikini Body Diet*, will also be amazing for your relationship (and your sex drive). Do each move for 1 minute, then repeat the entire circuit once or twice more.

Mirror Squat
Works butt and legs

- Stand facing each other, about a foot apart, with feet slightly wider than shoulders. Clasp each other's hands at chest height in front of you and squat until your thighs are parallel to the floor, then rise up to starting position.

Partner Press
Works shoulders, chest, triceps, and core

- Have your partner lie faceup with legs bent and feet on the floor. Get in plank position above him, with your hands on the floor beside your partner's shoulders; have him place his hands on your shoulders, elbows bent. Bend your elbows, and push up as your partner extends his arms, lifting you. Return to starting position and repeat for 30 seconds, then switch positions for the next 30.

Side Shuffle
Works butt and legs

- Stand facing each other with about a foot between you, feet hip-width apart. Bend elbows, raise arms to shoulder height in front of you, and press your palms against your partner's. Bend knees and step to the right as your partner steps to the left, then step back. Continue shuffling to the right for 30 seconds, then repeat in opposite direction.

Power Punch
Works shoulders, chest, and back

- Stand facing each other with feet staggered, left in front of right, and knees slightly bent. Hold your right hand at chest height in front of you, elbow bent; your partner extends his right arm. Clasp your right hand and place your left hand on your hips. Extend your right arm forward as your partner resists. Bend elbow and repeat for 15 seconds, then switch (partner punches and you resist) for 15 seconds. Repeat on opposite side.

Towel Twist
Works core, butt, and legs

- Hold a towel in front of your belly and stand facing away from your partner, feet shoulder-width apart and knees bent. Twist to the left as your partner twists to the right, and hand him the towel. Rotate to opposite side and grab the towel from your partner. Continue alternating sides and handing the towel to each other.

Pleasure to Meet You
Works shoulders, chest, and core

- Get in pushup position (either on toes or knees), head-to-head and about arm's length apart. Bend your elbows, lowering your chest toward the floor. Push up, lift right arm, and shake each other's hand. Return to starting position and repeat, this time shaking left hands. Continue, alternating hands on each rep.

Pull Together
Works back, abs, butt, and legs

- Lie faceup with knees bent and feet on the floor; your partner stands over your hips and squats. Extend your arms and grasp his left hand with your right, and his right with your left. Bend your elbows, pulling yourself toward your partner. Lower to starting position. Continue for 30 seconds, then switch positions, and repeat.

Rescue Me
Works shoulders, arms, back, and core

- Sit facing each other with knees bent and feet touching, each holding one end of a towel. Your partner lies faceup on the floor (the towel should be taut) and places his right hand above his left, then left above right, pulling himself up until he's sitting. Return to starting position and repeat for 30 seconds. Then switch positions (you lie down) and repeat.

High Five
Works entire body

- Lie faceup with knees bent and feet on the floor, toe-to-toe with your partner. Sit up as you place your left hand on the floor beside your left hip and extended your right arm in front of you, touching his right palm. Stand up, pushing against each other, jump, then high-five each other. Return to starting position and repeat with opposite hand.

Drum Line
Works shoulders, back, arms, butt, and legs

- Stand facing each other, about 2 feet apart, with feet wider than shoulders and knees bent. Your partner holds a towel taut at belly height horizontally in front of him. Bend elbows and bring your hands in front of your face, palms facing each other. "Chop" the towel with your left hand across the length for 15 seconds, then repeat with right hand for 15 seconds. Switch positions with your partner and repeat.

24-HOUR DAMAGE CONTROL

80 Ways to Kick Food Guilt to the Curb

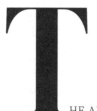

HE ALARM RINGS.

You reach one hand slowly, languidly toward the beckoning beacon, tap the snooze button, and roll back into your gauzy fantasy. It's you and Ryan Gosling, and he's feeding you ice cream. And dessert wine. And chocolate cake. *Oh no, Ryan, I couldn't possibly have another slice! And more wine...*

Wait. That was no dream. That was the random birthday party you wound up at last night. And that was no Ryan Gosling (although the guy did look a bit like a baby goose) ...

Panic. The food. The drink. The random dude. The more food! You set out to be a little bit Naughty, and somehow your night took a detour into the nasty. And now a neurotic brainstorming session ensues: How are you going to solve this? Two hours on the treadmill to burn off that dessert. Then one of those seven-day water cleanses. And you'll need to scrub all social media evidence . . . OMG! What did you Tweet? Surely a local Catholic church must offer exorcism by request . . .

Stop. We've all done this. I've done this. A metaphorical walk of shame–even if it's from your bedroom to your bathroom scale–is something every Naughty girl takes from time to time. What separates the truly Naughty from the rest of us is the ability to make mistakes and keep moving forward. Regrets are boring.

Self-forgiveness is the first rule of Naughty. Here's how you start facing the future:

1. **Take a 5-minute chill.** Breathe. Deeply. For five minutes.

2. **Open the blinds.** Put on sunglasses first, if you must. Morning rays help synchronize the body's internal clock that regulates circadian rhythms and metabolism, according to a study published in the journal *PLOS ONE*.[1] Just twenty to thirty minutes of morning light is enough to affect BMI, and even dim light with just half the intensity of sunlight on a cloudy day will do. Just put your clothes on first. Or not. Give the neighbors a show. You have nothing to hide.

3. **Look in the mirror.** Your body has already forgiven you. *You're not bad, you're just naughty.* Make peace. Naughty truce.

4. **Assume the power pose.** Stretch your arms out wide like you're crossing the finish line of the 100-yard dash. Amy Cuddy, social psychologist and professor at Harvard Business School, found people who assumed this pose for just two minutes experienced a decrease in cortisol (a hormone linked to fat gain) and an increased sense of power.[2] Chin up, boobs up. Open yourself up to the potential of a new, naughty, guilt-free day. You got this.

5. **Give yourself a big hug.** Research shows crossing your arms and giving yourself a tight squeeze can reduce physical pain.[3] Love up on the approximately 37.2 trillion cells that make up your naughty body.

6. **Master your mantra:** *I do enough. I am enough.* Research shows women who practice regular self-affirmation have less body dissatisfaction and a greater intention of reducing criticism of their body.[4] (Flip back to page 28 for some naughty favorites.)

7. **Rehydrate.** Whatever nastiness went down last night, it probably threw off your antidiuretic hormones–the chemicals that control how much water you hold on to. (Salt and alcohol are major culprits.) If you look in the mirror and see someone who gained weight overnight, it's an illusion: You're probably just retaining water. It sounds illogical, but the best way to lose that water weight quickly is to start rehydrating. Fill up a large pitcher of iced water with three to four sliced lemons. Citrus fruits are rich in the antioxidant de-limonene, a powerful compound found in the peel that stimulates liver enzymes to help flush toxins from the body, according to the World Health Organization.[5] Have a tall glass now, fill a water bottle to sip on throughout the day, and keep a pitcher in the fridge. German researchers found that six cups of cold water a day could prompt a metabolic boost that incinerates 50 daily calories. That's enough to shed 5 pounds a year!

8. **Destroy any circumstantial evidence.** Throw out any empty food packaging. Hoover any crumbs. Mop up any spills. Fill the dishwasher. The faster you mop up the physical evidence, the faster you'll clean up the emotional detritus.

9. **Hide your binge triggers.** A study by Google found that placing candies in opaque containers as opposed to glass ones curbed candy consumption by 3.1 million calories among their employees in just seven weeks.[6] If it works on geeks, it will work on you: Move any binge-worthy foods to the high shelves and shut the door. Out of sight, out of mouth.

10. Shut your food window. Today, we're skipping breakfast. Yes, it's the most important meal of the day–if you're in kindergarten. But for grown-ups, it makes sense to build in calorie-free periods of 12 to 16 hours for every 24. This technique, known as intermittent fasting–or reducing your "eating window"–can help to reset your metabolism and burn the extra glucose (sugar/carbs) in your system after a period of overindulgence, according to a study in the journal *Cell Metabolism*.[7] And a recent study at the University of Southern California found that doing this just four days in a row every two weeks can reduce belly fat and slow aging.[8] NOTE: This isn't about restricting calories; Naughty girls never restrict calories. Instead, it's about letting your digestive system heal and recover so it can bring its best to the table.

11. Have some green tea. A recent Taiwanese study found that one to two cups of green tea before breakfast can improve metabolism, helping you burn off additional calories–and whatever else is hanging around your system from last night.[9]

12. Remember, what worries you, masters you. Make Food Guilt your bitch. Reread Chapter 4, if you need to. Write down what you regret, then tear it up and flush it. #sorrynotsorry.

13. Make today Throwback Thursday. Hating on yourself still? Break that cycle! Look at cute pics of yourself as a kid. Would you ever be as hard on that little munchkin as you are on yourself? Tell her everything is okay. Because it is.

14. F*&#% FOOD GUILT! Swearing in public is not cool, but in the privacy of your own home? It might be your secret weapon: One study found that swearing is not only a harmless emotional release (as long as you're not swearing at someone), but it can actually make you feel stronger.[10] Eff yeah!

15. Do NOT weigh yourself. Yes, the needle might budge a bit upward, but that's not because you've actually gained weight. What would happen if you slammed your hand in a door? It would swell. You wouldn't think, *Oh shit, my hand is going to look like a baseball mitt forever.* Your body reacts to a food binge just as it would another injury. See your bloat as a sign of healing. All will be gone in a few hours. Weigh-ins are for wrestlers.

16. I repeat: Do NOT weigh yourself. To gain one legit pound of fat in a day you would have to eat 3,500 calories *more* than what you burned off. Since the average woman burns 1,600 calories a day just sitting around, you would have to eat a total of 5,100 calories to add just 1 pound of fat to your frame overnight. That means you'd have to eat twenty-two large slices of Domino's thin-crust cheese pizzas, or drink 8.5 bottles of wine. (Don't get any ideas).

17. Take a cold shower. Or at least, end with a cold blast. In a study at Kentucky State, researchers found that exposure to cold temperatures for five minutes in the morning stimulated brown fat cells, increasing the rate at which you burn calories throughout the day.[11] A second study found that the action of warming your body back up after a cold immersion forces you into a state of calm.[12]

18. And sing while you do. Food Guilt cannot exist in a happy, positive environment. Who's walking on sunshine now?

19. Turn up the chill. Listen to the song "Weightless" by Marconi Union while you get ready. According to a study conducted by Mindlab International Ltd., it is the most relaxing song ever recorded.[13]

20. Dress beautifully. I know, you're battling shame and all you want is that ratty U. of Wisconsin hoodie. But not today, My Naughty. Wear something beautiful, sophisticated, feminine, and polished. With your sexiest lingerie underneath. Research shows people describe themselves in a way that's consistent with how they are dressed.[14] Dress the part, feel the part. Save the bulky clothes for a day when your confidence is running high.

21. Choose low or moderate heels. If you feel wobbly, you'll be wobbly. Avoid looking like a baby giraffe and leave the 4-inch strappies at home today.

22. Wear perfume. A study published in the *Journal of Cosmetic Sciences* found that people who spritzed with cologne experienced a boost in both self-confidence and self-perceived attractiveness.[15]

23. Walk to work. Or take the stairs once you're there. Take advantage of your calorie-free morning and comfortable shoes by walking a little more than you ordinarily might. Moving around before you eat means any energy you burn comes right from your fat stores instead of the glucose (sugar) still in your system. According to some studies, exercising in a fasted state can burn almost 20 percent more fat than exercising with fuel in the tank.[16]

24. Smile at a stranger. And another one. According to a 2012 study from the University of Kansas, smiling during stressful situations can help ease anxiety–even if you don't feel happy.[17] Grin and bear it.

25. Juke the jitters. A study found *decaffeinated* coffee resulted in significantly lower hunger levels and higher plasma levels of PYY (an appetite-suppressing hormone) than caffeinated beverages.[18]

26. Shut your Facebook. A study found that as social media interaction increased, self-esteem decreased–especially among female users, who were more apt to feel unhappy with their lives than men.[19]

27. After you post something great. A team of researchers found that people with high self-esteem spend more time adding information about their family, education, and work experience; while users with a lower self-esteem are more likely to monitor their walls like a hawk and delete all unwanted posts from other users.[20] Remember, it's your story. Don't let anybody else write it!

28. Steal the future. Pick your favorite horoscope and pretend it's your own. Hey, it's a victimless crime!

29. Put in your headphones and get to work. A study by Penn State University found students who listened to music–almost any type– reported feeling more optimistic, calm and relaxed.[21] To transport your- self back to Mojito Beach, you gotta go with some reggae. That means the father of reggae: Mr. Marley; or, for something more up tempo and dirtier: Sean Paul.

30. Keep drinking! Make sure you've had at least two large glasses of spa water before noon. A study in the *Journal of Clinical Endocrinology and Metabolism* found just 17 ounces of water increased participants' meta- bolic rates by 30 percent.[22]

31. Take your karma in for a tune-up. Pay a female co-worker a genu- ine compliment that has absolutely nothing to do with her looks.

32. Moisturize. Give yourself a hand massage with some luxurious lotion. A recent study found that a five-minute hand massage significantly low- ered stress levels.[23]

33. Take a brief exercise break. If you can't do a full workout, then do some light stretching and punctuate it with quick, hard-working fitness bursts. Research printed in the journal *Physiological Reports* showed that people who did five thirty-second bursts of max-effort exercise, burned 200 extra calories that day–not that we're counting.[24]

34. Become a Greek goddess. Once you're safely past your belly-healing window, consider kicking into your day of eating healthy with some Greek yogurt. It's creamy–which will cater to any emotional need for comfort–and packed with protein. A recent study in the *FASEB Jour- nal* showed that high-protein breakfasts help maintain blood sugar and insulin levels far better than no-protein meals.[25] And after last night's mega spike, steady and stable is exactly what we want.

35. Slice a banana on top. It's one of the best natural sources of vitamin B_6, which research shows can reduce hangover symptoms by as much as 50 percent![26]

36. But not too ripe. Firm bananas are healthier because they're higher in resistant starch, which helps feed the healthy bacteria in your gut.

37. Watch a grumpy cat video on YouTube. A recent study found watching cat videos can boost feelings of happiness and moderate guilt.[27]

38. Postpone your snacks. Snacking is a beautiful thing, but resist the urge until after lunch. A study in the *Journal of the American Dietetic Association* found that morning snackers tend to eat more throughout the day than afternoon snackers.[28]

39. Pop a mint or a stick of gum. The minty scent helps to relax and relieve headaches, and has the added bonus as a proven appetite suppressant. One study in the *Journal of Neurological and Orthopedic Medicine* found that people who sniffed peppermint every two hours lost an average of 5 pounds a month.[29]

40. Make a fist. The kindly matron down in sales brought all the leftover cookies from a client meeting around for the staff to enjoy. Find the power to resist: A study published in the *Journal of Consumer Research* found people who tightened their muscles, regardless of which ones–hand, finger, calf, or biceps–while trying to exercise self-control were better able to resist temptation.[30] Clench your hand, clench your jaw, smile, and say no.

41. Plan an indulgence. You're not about sacrifices, Naughty girl! You're just making today extra healthy. Make a dinner reservation at your favorite restaurant for next weekend.

42. Take a salad break. Make it a spinach one with lots of colorful veggie toppings. The meal will flood your system with the vitamins and antioxidants it needs to heal; plus a recent Swedish study suggests compounds in the leaf membranes, called thylakoids, may serve as a powerful appetite suppressant.[31]

43. Add some avocado. The monounsaturated fats will help your body to absorb the fat-soluble nutrient in the salad, plus research suggests the creamy fruit may help spot-reduce belly fat.[32]

44. Van Gogh, girl! Pop into a museum for ten minutes. Or just image search some beautiful works (artnet.com is a great resource). A recent University College of London experiment found that looking at artwork can trigger the same pleasure responses in the brain as falling in love.[33] Oh happy day!

45. Take a Funny or Die break. You just burned 40 to 170 calories, according to a study published in the *International Journal of Obesity* that suggests genuine laughter may cause a 10 to 20 percent increase in resting metabolism.[34]

46. Sext your darling at work.

47. Yawn. Release a tunnel of pent-up energy and send a blast of vitamin O to the brain.

48. Snack on a red grapefruit. A study in the journal *Metabolism* found that eating half a grapefruit before meals may help reduce belly fat; participants in a six-week study who ate grapefruit with every meal saw their waist shrink by up to an inch.[35]

49. Or anything red or orange. Carotenoids, the vitamins that give orange and red fruits their color, give your skin a sun-kissed glow from the inside. Studies show that observers prefer the coloring that comes from carotenoids more than they do an actual suntan.[36] The preventing cancer thing is just a bonus.

50. Plan a sexy vacation. A study published in the journal *Applied Research in Quality of Life* showed that the highest spike in happiness came during the planning stage of a vacation as people enjoy the sense of anticipation.[37]

51. Do a posture check. Imagine a string attached to the top of your head, pulling it up toward the sky. If you're standing, make sure your ears, shoulders, hips, knees, and ankles are aligned. Better breathing and a sense of confidence are your reward, and maybe a cleaner internal engine. A study in the appropriately titled journal *Gut* found that being upright was much more effective in reducing intestinal gas retention than lying down on the back.[38] Posture, the researchers say, has a big influence on the movement of gas through the system.

52. Walk home.

53. Skip!

54. Stop and buy yourself a dozen roses.

55. Draw yourself a hot bath. One study found that submerging in hot water can be as good for the heart as plodding away on the *dreadmill*, as the hot temperature increases the volume of blood pumping to and from the organ.[39] See page 191 for my recipe for a truly decadent bath.

56. Exfoliate. Shave your legs. Slough off that old skin!

57. Apply some vacation. Massage your gorgeous gams with a generous dollop of high-quality coconut-scented body butter. Breathe in the tropical scent and imagine you're back on Mojito Beach and a sexy man is lathering you up. Research shows the scent of coconut can relieve stress.[40]

58. Love yourself. While you're massaging your legs, let your hands wander upward a bit. A little self-love can trigger the release of oxytocin, the "love hormone" naturally released during sex, that can minimize stress hormones and suppress the appetite, according to a study in the journal *Aging*.[41] What's more, research shows women who masturbate have greater self-esteem than their nonmasturbating counterparts.[42] As if you needed another reason to hit the naughty drawer.

59. Take it to the top. Orgasm promotes relaxation, according to a white paper by Planned Parenthood.[43] And since you're solo you don't even need to think about anything Planned Parenthood related. O-yeah.

60. Slip into something sexy and comfortable. No Juicy sweatpants allowed. Quality, quality, quality. You are a Queen, not a couch pillow. No velour, ever!

61. Toast your victory. You've vanquished Food Guilt for another day. Assuming you're not hungover, pour yourself a glass of red. One compound, ellagic acid, has been shown to change the way "fat genes" express themselves, boosting the metabolism and slowing the growth of existing and new fat cells.[44] More research suggests another healthy ingredient in wine–resveratrol–could help to counter some of the negative effects associated with lack of exercise, like muscle-loss and blood sugar sensitivities.[45]

62. Dim the dinner lights. Pull out the candelabra and put on some Barry White. Put your roses on the table. A study in the journal *Psychological Reports* found people eat about 175 fewer calories when dining in a relaxed environment with dimmed lights and mellow music.[46]

63. Prepare a beautiful, colorful, SOUL food meal. Try my Brick Lane Curry on page 145.

64. Double down on greens. Research from the University of Otago found that participants felt happier, calmer, and more positive on days when they consumed fruits and vegetables.[47]

65. Grind off the pounds. Finish the dish with freshly ground black pepper. Research suggests piperine, the compound that gives the spice its characteristic kick, may have the profound ability to decrease inflammation and block the formation of new fat cells.[48] Freshly ground pepper is higher in the compound than the stale old stuff in the shaker.

66. Practice tantric eating. Minimize distractions. Turn off the TV, put down your phone, close the laptop. Engage with your food and let it engage with you.

67. Take a knife to it. Experts say gauging your body's subtle "I'm full" cues is easier when you take smaller bites at a slower pace. People eat up to 25 percent less when their food is cut into small pieces, according to an Arizona State University study.[49]

68. Play food critic. After each bite, list a new adjective to describe the taste, look, scent, and mouthfeel of your meal. Appreciation up, face-stuffing down.

69. Go for an evening stroll. One study found walking at a leisurely pace after eating a meal helped food move through the stomach much more quickly than an espresso or alcoholic digestif.[50]

70. Look up at the moon. Pause to take in the natural wonder. How pretty your guilt looks in the reflection of moonlight.

71. Snack on the dark side. A recent study from Louisiana State University found that gut microbes in our stomach ferment chocolate in a way that helps to reduce inflammation and fat storage.[51] Look for a cacao percentage of 70 or above.

72. Turn down the thermostat. A new study suggests that simply turning on the AC can stimulate fat burning.[52] Another study by the American Meteorological Society found that happiness is maximized at 57 degrees.[53]

73. Stretch. Pennsylvania researchers found practicing gentle yoga for as little as twenty minutes daily banishes insomnia as effectively as sleeping pills![54]

74. Brew up some exotic herbals. Consider the rarely used ashwagandha tea. A study in the *Indian Journal of Psychological Medicine* found that "ashwagandha root extract safely and effectively improves an individual's resistance toward stress and thereby improves self-assessed quality of life."[55] In another study, serum cortisol levels in a group of ashwagandha drinkers were substantially reduced versus a placebo group.[56] The plant is used in traditional Ayurvedic medicine to treat nervous exhaustion, insomnia and loss of memory.

75. Turn off your phone. And your laptop. And iPad, too. Research shows that exposure to artificial light, especially LED blue light like your electronic screens, before bedtime suppresses levels of melatonin–the hormone that regulates natural sleep cycles.[57]

76. Take a trip to Provence. Put a few drops of lavender oil on your pillow. Research shows the Provençal scent serves as a mild sedative and can increase the percentage of slow, deep sleep waves.[58]

77. Move the roses to your bedside table. A recent study found people exposed to the rose scent while sleeping reported rosier dreams.[59]

78. Get to bed early. Getting seven to nine hours of sleep is one of the best things you can do to get back on track after a binge. In a University of Colorado study, participants who were only permitted to sleep a mere five hours ate more the next day than those who got nine hours of shut-eye.[60]

79. Count your blessings. You are blessed. You are loved. You are sleepy...

80. Close your eyes. Dream of something naughty . . . tomorrow is another day, my Naughty.

NOTES

Step 1
Embrace the Four Naughty Mantras

1. S. Basu, P. Yoffe, N. Hills, and R. H. Lustig, "The Relationship of Sugar to Population-Level Diabetes Prevalence: An Econometric Analysis of Repeated Cross-Sectional Data," *PLOS ONE* 8, no. 2 (2013): e57873, doi: 10.1371/journal.pone.0057873.

2. S. C. Lucan and J. J. DiNicolantonio, "How Calorie-Focused Thinking About Obesity and Related Diseases May Mislead and Harm Public Health: An Alternative," *Public Health Nutrition* 19, no. 4 (March 2015): 571–81, doi: 10.1017/S1368980014002559, published electronically November 24, 2014, PubMed PMID: 25416919.

3. J. A. L. Calbet, J. G. Ponce-González, I. Pérez-Suárez, J. de la Calle Herrero, and H.-C. Holmberg, "A Time-Efficient Reduction of Fat Mass in 4 Days with Exercise and Caloric Restriction," *Scandinavian Journal of Medicine & Science in Sports* 25 (2015): 223–33, doi: 10.1111/sms.12194.

4. M. D. Mozaffarian, T. Hao, E. B. Rimm, W. C. Willett, and F. B. Hu, "Changes in Diet and Lifestyle and Long-Term Weight Gain in Women and Men," *New England Journal of Medicine* 364 (2011): 2392–2404.

5. C. E. Adams and M. R. Leary, "Promoting Self-Compassionate Attitudes Toward Eating Among Restrictive and Guilty Eaters," *Journal of Social and Clinical Psychology* 26 (2007): 1120–44.

6. J. Wardle, A. Steptoe, G. Oliver, and Z. Lipsey, "Stress, Dietary Restraint and Food Intake," *Journal of Psychosomatic Research* 48, no. 2 (February 2000): 195–202, published electronically, PubMed PMID: 10719137.

Step 3
Stop the Shame Game

1. "Ashley Judd: Puffy Face Controversy 'Really Isn't About Me,'" NBC *Rock Center with Brian Williams*, April 11, 2012. nbcnews.com

2. Lindsay Cronin, "Giuliana Rancic Instagram: E! News Host Criticized for Being Too Thin After Sharing New Photo," EnStars, March 27, 2015. enstar2.com

3. C. J. Ferguson, M. E. Muñoz, A. Garza, and M. Galindo, "Concurrent and Prospective Analyses of Peer, Television and Social Media Influences on Body Dissatisfaction, Eating Disorder Symptoms and Life Satisfaction in Adolescent Girls," *Journal of Youth and Adolescence* 43, no. 1 (January 2014): 1–14, doi: 10.1007/s10964-012-9898-9.

4. R. Engeln and R. H. Salk, "The Demographics of Fat Talk in Adult Women: Age, Body Size, and Ethnicity," *Journal of Health Psychology* (December 8, 2014), p ii: 1359105314560918, published electronically, PubMed PMID: 25488938.

5. J. F. Benenson, "The Development of Human Female Competition: Allies and Adversaries," *Philosophical Transactions of the Royal Society: Biological Sciences* 368, no. 1631 (October 28, 2013): 20130079, doi: 10.1098/rstb.2013.0079, published electronically, PubMed PMID: 24167309, review published electronically, PubMed Central PMCID: PMC3826208.

6. A. L. Meltzer, J. K. McNulty, S. L. Miller, and L. R. Baker, "A Psychophysiological Mechanism Underlying Women's Weight-Management Goals: Women Desire and Strive for Greater Weight Loss Near Peak Fertility," *Personality and Social Psychology Bulletin* 41, no. 7 (July 2015): 930-42, doi: 10.1177/0146167215585726.

7. A.L. Orsama, E. Mattila, M. Ermes, M. van Gils, B. Wansink, and I. Korhonen, "Weight Rhythms: Weight Increases During Weekends and Decreases During Weekdays," *Obesity Facts* 7 (2014): 36-47.

8. Melissa Milne, "I Eat Slim-Shamers for Breakfast," Yahoo! Health, April 7, 2015.yahoo.com

Step 4
Make Guilt Your Bitch

1. I. Etxebarria, M. J. Ortiz, S. Conejero, and A. Pascual, "Intensity of Habitual Guilt in Men and Women: Differences in Interpersonal Sensitivity and the Tendency Towards Anxious-Aggressive Guilt," *Spanish Journal of Psychology* 12, no. 2 (November 2009): 540-54.

2. R. G. Kuijer and J. A. Boyce, "Chocolate Cake. Guilt or Celebration? Associations with Healthy Eating Attitudes, Perceived Behavioural Control, Intentions and Weight-Loss," *Appetite* 74 (March 2014): 48-54, doi: 10.1016/j.appet.2013.11.013, published electronically November 13, 2013, PubMed PMID: 24275670.

3. J. P. Tangney, J. Stuewig, and A. G. Martinez, "Two Faces of Shame: The Roles of Shame and Guilt in Predicting Recidivism," *Psychological Science* 25, no. 3 (March 2014): 799-805, doi: 10.1177/0956797613508790.

Step 5
Listen to Your Body

1. Danci et al., "Low-Carbohydrate Weight-Loss Diets. Effects on Cognition and Mood," *Appetite*, 52, no. 1 (2009): 96, doi: 10.1016/j.appet.2008.08.009.

2. B. J. Bushman, C. N. Dewall, R. S. Pond Jr., and M. D. Hanus, "Low Glucose Relates to Greater Aggression in Married Couples," *Proceedings of the National Academy of Sciences of the United States of America* 111, no. 17 (April 29, 2014): 6254-57, doi: 10.1073/pnas.1400619111.

3. E. M. Schulte, N. M. Avena, and A. N. Gearhardt, "Which Foods May Be Addictive? The Roles of Processing, Fat Content, and Glycemic Load," *PLOS ONE* 10, no. 2 (February 18, 2015): e0117959, doi: 10.1371/journal.pone.0117959, eCollection 2015, PubMed PMID: 25692302, PubMed Central PMCID: PMC4334652.

4. F. McKiernan, J. A. Houchins, and R. D. Mattes, "Relationships Between Human Thirst, Hunger, Drinking, and Feeding," *Physiology & Behavior* 94, no. 5 (2008): 700–708, doi: 10.1016/j.physbeh.2008.04.007.

5. M. Sato, M. Murakami, K. Node, R. Matsumura, and M. Akashi, "The Role of the Endocrine System in Feeding-Induced Tissue-Specific Circadian Entrainment," *Cell Reports* 8, no. 2 (July 24, 2014): 393–401, doi: 10.1016/j.celrep.2014.06.015.

Step 6
Find Your P-Spot

1. H. Brown, "Go with Your Gut," *New York Times*, February 20, 2006.

2. J. McQuaid, "The Science of Mmm: How Food and Drink Tickle the Brain's Pleasure Centers," *Slate*, January 22, 2015.

3. D. Jakubowicz, O. Froy, J. Wainstein, and M. Boaz, "Meal Timing and Composition Influence Ghrelin Levels, Appetite Scores and Weight Loss Maintenance in Overweight and Obese Adults," *Steroids* 77, no. 4 (March 10, 2012): 323–31, doi: 10.1016/j. steroids.2011.12.006, published electronically December 9, 2012, erratum in *Steroids* 77, no. 8–9 (July 2012): 887–89, PubMed PMID: 22178258.

4. L. A. Latimer, L. Pope, and B. Wansink, "Food Neophiles: Profiling the Adventurous Eater," *Obesity* (Silver Spring) 23, no. 8 (August 2015): 1577–81, doi: 10.1002/oby.21154.

5. M. D. Mozaffarian, T. Hao, E. B. Rimm, W. C. Willett, and B. B. Hu, "Changes in Diet and Lifestyle and Long-Term Weight Gain in Women and Men," *New England Journal of Medicine* 364 (2011): 2392–2404.

6. M. M. Hetherington and J. I. Macdiarmid, "Pleasure and Excess: Liking for and Over-consumption of Chocolate," *Psychology & Behavior* 57, no. 1 (January 1995): 27–35, PubMed PMID: 7878121.

7. T. L. Davidson, A. A. Martin, K. Clark, and S. E. Swithers, "Intake of High-Intensity Sweeteners Alters the Ability of Sweet Taste to Signal Caloric Consequences: Implications for the Learned Control of Energy and Body Weight Regulation," *Quarterly Journal of Experimental Psychology* (2006) 64, no. 7 (2011): 1430–41, doi: 10.1080/17470218.2011.552729.

8. S. P. Fowler, K. Williams, and H. P. Hazuda, "Diet Soda Intake Is Associated with Long-Term Increases in Waist Circumference in a Biethnic Cohort of Older Adults: The San Antonio Longitudinal Study of Aging," *Journal of the American Geriatrics Society* 63, no. 4 (April 2015): 708–15, doi: 10.1111/jgs.13376.

9. M. E. Bocarsly, E. S. Powell, N. M. Avena, and B. G. Hoebel, "High-Fructose Corn Syrup Causes Characteristics of Obesity in Rats: Increased Body Weight, Body Fat and Triglyceride Levels," *Pharmacology Biochemistry and Behavior* 97, no. 1 (November 2010): 101–6, doi: 10.1016/j.pbb.2010.02.012.

10. T. A. Judge and D. M. Cable, "When It Comes to Pay, Do the Thin Win? The Effect of Weight on Pay for Men And Women," *Journal of Applied Psychology* 96, no. 1 (January 2011): 95–112, doi: 10.1037/a0020860.

11. K. D. Vohs, Y. Wang, F. Gino, and M. I. Norton, "Rituals Enhance Consumption," *Psychological Science* 24, no. 9 (September 2013): 1714–21, doi: 10.1177/0956797613478949, published electronically July 17, 2013, PubMed PMID: 23863754.a.

12. R. G. Kuijer and J. A. Boyce, "Chocolate Cake. Guilt or Celebration? Associations with Healthy Eating Attitudes, Perceived Behavioural Control, Intentions and Weight-Loss," *Appetite* 74 (March 2014): 48–54, doi: 10.1016/j.appet.2013.11.013, published electronically November 23, 2013, PubMed PMID: 24275670.

13. R. A. De Wijk, I. A. Polet, W. Boek, S. Coenraad, and J. H. F. Bult, "Food Aroma Affects Bite Size," *Flavour*, (March 2012), doi: 10.1186/2044-7248-1-3.

14. Brian Wansink, *Slim by Design: Mindless Eating Solutions for Everyday Life* (New York: Morrow, 2014).

15. B. Wansink and K. van Ittersum, "Fast Food Restaurant Lighting and Music Can Reduce Calorie Intake and Increase Satisfaction," *Psychological Reports* 111, no. 1 (August 2012): 228–32, PubMed PMID: 23045865.

16. C. K. Morewedge, Y. E. Huh, and J. Vosgerau, "Thought for Food: Imagined Consumption Reduces Actual Consumption," *Science* 330, no. 6010 (December 10, 2010): 1530–33, doi: 10.1126/science.1195701, PubMed PMID: 21148388.

17. C. Michel, C. Velasco, and C. Spence, "A Taste of Kandinsky: Assessing the Influence of the Artistic Visual Presentation of Food on the Dining Experience," *Flavour*, (June 2014), doi: 10.1186/2044-7248-3-7.

Step 7
Eat Naughty Foods

1. C. A. Daley, A. Abbott, P. S. Doyle, G. A. Nader, and S. Larson, "A Review of Fatty Acid Profiles and Antioxidant Content in Grass-Fed and Grain-Fed Beef," *Nutrition Journal* 9 (March 19, 2010): 10, doi: 10.1186/1475-2891-9-10, review PubMed PMID: 20219103, PubMed Central PMCID: PMC2846864.

2. K. E. Nachman, P. A. Baron, G. Raber, K. A. Francesconi, A. Navas-Acien, and D. C. Love, "Roxarsone, Inorganic Arsenic, and Other Arsenic Species in Chicken: A U.S.-Based Market Basket Sample," *Environmental Health Perspectives* 121, no. 7 (July 2013): 818–24, doi: 10.1289/ehp.1206245.

3. F. A. Guarraci and A. Benson, "'Coffee, Tea and Me': Moderate Doses of Caffeine Affect Sexual Behavior in Female Rats," *Pharmacology Biochemistry and Behavior* 82, no. 3 (November 2005): 522–30.

4. N. Mondaini, T. Cai, P. Gontero, A. Gavazzi, G. Lombardi, V. Boddi, and R. Bartoletti, "Regular Moderate Intake of Red Wine Is Linked to a Better Women's Sexual Health," *Journal of Sexual Medicine* 6, no. 10 (October 2009): 2772–77, doi: 10.1111/j.1743-6109.2009.01393.x, published electronically July 21, 2009, PubMed PMID: 19627470.

Step 9
Chill the Eff Out

1. A.R. Hirsch and R. Gomez, "Weight Reduction Through Inhalation of Odorants," *Journal of Neurological and Orthopaedic Medicine and Surgery* 16 (1995): 26–31.

2. C. K. Morewedge, Y. E. Huh, and J. Vosgerau, "Thought for Food: Imagined Consumption Reduces Actual Consumption," *Science* 330, no. 6010 (December 10, 2010): 1530–33, doi: 10.1126/science.1195701, PubMed PMID: 21148388.

3. S. E. Jackson, A. Steptoe, and J. Wardle, "The Influence of Partner's Behavior on Health Behavior Change: The English Longitudinal Study of Ageing," *JAMA Internal Medicine* 175, no. 3 (March 2015): 385–92, doi: 10.1001/jamainternmed.2014.7554, PubMed PMID: 25599511.

4. J. C. Rickman, D. M. Barrett, and C. M. Bruhn, "Nutritional Comparison of Fresh, Frozen and Canned Fruits and Vegetables, Part 1: Vitamins C and B and Phenolic Compounds," *Journal of the Science of Food and Agriculture* 87 (2007): 930–44, doi: 10.1002/jsfa.2825.

5. C. J. Rebello, Y.-F. Chu, W. D. Johnson, et al., "The Role of Meal Viscosity and Oat-glucan Characteristics in Human Appetite Control: A Randomized Crossover Trial," *Nutrition Journal* 13 (2014): 49, doi: 10.1186/1475-2891-13-49.

6. Texas A&M AgriLife Communications, "Peaches, Plums, Nectarines Give Obesity, Diabetes Slim Chance," *ScienceDaily*, June 18, 2012.

7. J. E. Flood-Obbagy and B. J. Rolls, "The Effect of Fruit in Different Forms on Energy Intake and Satiety at a Meal," *Appetite* 52, no. 2 (2009): 416–22, doi: 10.1016/j.appet.2008.12.001.

8. A. V. Nedeltcheva, J. M. Kilkus, J. Imperial, et al., "Insufficient Sleep Undermines Dietary Efforts to Reduce Adiposity," *Annals of Internal Medicine* 153 (2010): 435–41a, doi: 10.7326/0003-4819-153-7-201010050-00006, PubMed PMID: 20921542.

9. S. Taheri, "The Link Between Short Sleep Duration and Obesity: We Should Recommend More Sleep to Prevent Obesity," *Archives of Disease in Childhood* 91, no. 11 (2006): 881–84, doi: 10.1136/adc.2005.093013.

10. Nedeltcheva et al., "Insufficient Sleep."

11. E. Hartmann and C. L. Spinweber, "Sleep Induced by L-tryptophan. Effect of Dosages Within the Normal Dietary Intake," *Journal of Nervous and Mental Disease* 167, no. 8 (August 1979): 497–99, PubMed PMID: 469515.

12. R. R. Markwald, E. L. Melanson, M. R. Smith, et al., "Impact of Insufficient Sleep on Total Daily Energy Expenditure, Food Intake, and Weight Gain," *Proceedings of the National Academy of Sciences of the United States of America* 110, no. 44 (2013): 5695–5700, doi: 10.1073/pnas.1216951110.

13. M. Hatori, C. Vollmers, A. Zarrinpar, et al., "Time Restricted Feeding Without Reducing Caloric Intake Prevents Metabolic Diseases in Mice Fed a High Fat Diet," *Cell Metabolism* 15, no. 6 (2012): 848–60, doi: 10.1016/j.cmet.2012.04.019.

14. T. A. Madzima, L. B. Panton, S. K. Fretti, A. W. Kinsey, and M. J. Ormsbee, "Night-time Consumption of Protein or Carbohydrate Results in Increased Morning Resting Energy Expenditure in Active College-Aged Men," *British Journal of Nutrition* 111, no. 1 (January 14, 2014): 71–77, doi: 10.1017/S000711451300192X, published electronically June 17, 2013, PubMed PMID: 23768612.

15. Hirsch and Gomez, "Weight Reduction."

16. P. Lee, S. Smith, J. Linderman, A. B. Courville, R. J. Brychta, W. Dieckmann, C. D. Werner, K. Y. Chen, and F. S. Celi, "Temperature-Acclimated Brown Adipose Tissue Modulates Insulin Sensitivity in Humans," *Diabetes.* 63, no. 11 (November 2014): 3686–98, doi: 10.2337/db14-0513, published electronically June 22, 2014, PubMed PMID: 24954193, PubMed Central PMCID: PMC4207391.

17. E. McFadden, M. E. Jones, M. J. Schoemaker, A. Ashworth, and A. J. Swerdlow, "The Relationship Between Obesity and Exposure to Light at Night: Cross-Sectional Analyses of over 100,000 Women in the Breakthrough Generations Study," *American Journal of Epidemiology* 180, no. 3 (August 1, 2014): 245–50, doi: 10.1093/aje/kwu117, published electronically May 29, 2014, PubMed PMID: 24875371.

18. "The Surprising Reason You're Gaining Weight," *Eat This, Not That!.* eatthis.com

19. H. Chahal, C. Fung, S. Kuhle, and P. J. Veugelers, "Availability and Night-time Use of Electronic Entertainment and Communication Devices Are Associated with Short Sleep Duration and Obesity Among Canadian Children," *Journal of Pediatric Obesity* 8, no. 1 (February 2013: 42–51, doi: 10.1111/j.2047-6310.2012.00085.x, published electronically September 7, 2012, PubMed PMID: 22962067.

20. T. G. Allison, T. D. Miller, R. W. Squires, and G. T. Gau, "Cardiovascular Responses to Immersion in a Hot Tub in Comparison with Exercise in Male Subjects with Coronary Artery Disease," *Mayo Clinic Proceedings* 68, no. 1 (January 1993): 19–25, PubMed PMID: 8417250.

21. P. L. Hooper, "Hot-tub Therapy for Type 2 Diabetes Mellitus," *New England Journal of Medicine* 341, no. 12 (September 16, 1999: 924–25, PubMed PMID: 10498473.

22. M. Flechtner-Mors, H. K. Biesalski, C. P. Jenkinson, G. Adler, and H. H. Ditschuneit, "Effects of Moderate Consumption of White Wine on Weight Loss in Overweight and Obese Subjects," *International Journal of Obesity Related Metabolic Disorders* 28, no. 11 (November 2004): 1420–26, PubMed PMID: 15356671.

Step 10
Change Your Brain, Change Your Body

1. L. Stahre and T. Hallstrom, "A Short-Term Cognitive Group Treatment Program Gives Substantial Weight Reduction up to 18 Months from the End of Treatment: A Randomized Controlled Trial," *Eating and Weight Disorders* 10 (2005): 51–58.

2. K. C. Maki, M. S. Reeves, M. Farmer, K. Yasunaga, N. Matsuo, Y. Katsuragi, M. Komikado, I. Tokimitsu, D. Wilder, F. Jones, J. B. Blumberg, and Y. Cartwright, "Green Tea Catechin Consumption Enhances Exercise-Induced Abdominal Fat Loss in Overweight and Obese Adults," *Journal of Nutrition* 139, no. 2 (February 2009): 264–70, doi: 10.3945/jn.108.098293, published electronically December 11, 2008, PubMed PMID: 19074207.

3. J. T. Gonzalez, R. C. Veasey, P. L. Rumbold, and E. J. Stevenson, "Breakfast and Exercise Contingently Affect Postprandial Metabolism and Energy Balance in Physically Active Males," *British Journal of Nutrition* 110, no. 4 (August 2013): 721–32, doi: 10.1017/S0007114512005582. published electronically January 29, 2013, PubMed PMID: 23340006.

4. K. J. Sevits, E. L. Melanson, T. Swibas, et al., "Total Daily Energy Expenditure Is Increased Following a Single Bout of Sprint Interval Training," *Physiological Reports* 1, no. 5 (2013): e00131, doi: 10.1002/phy2.131.

5. G. Charness and U. Gneezy, "Incentives to Exercise," *Econometrica* 77 (2009): 909–31, doi: 10.3982/ECTA7416

6. K. A. Martin Ginis, M. E. Jung, and L. Gauvin, "To See or Not To See: Effects of Exercising in Mirrored Environments on Sedentary Women's Feeling States and Self-Efficacy," *Health Psychology* 22, no. 4 (July 2003: 354–61, PubMed PMID: 12940391.

7. Y. H. Kee and C. K. J. Wang, "Relationships Between Mindfulness, Flow Dispositions and Mental Skills Adoption: A Cluster Analytic Approach," *Psychology of Sport and Exercise* 9 (2008): 393–411.

8. Alia J. Crum and Ellen J. Langer, "Mind-set Matters: Exercise and the Placebo Effect," *Psychological Science* 18, no. 2 (2007): 165–71.

9. Jeremy D. Goldhaber-Fiebert, Erik Blumenkranz, and Alan M. Garber, *Committing to Exercise: Contract Design for Virtuous Habit Formation* (Cambridge, MA: National Bureau of Economic Research, ca. 2010).

10. B. Prabhakaran, E. A. Dowling, J. D. Branch, D. P. Swain, and B. C. Leutholtz, "Effect of 14 Weeks of Resistance Training on Lipid Profile and Body Fat Percentage in Premenopausal Women," *British Journal of Sports Medicine* 33, no. 3 (June 1999): 190–95, PubMed PMID: 10378072, PubMed Central PMCID: PMC1756170.

11. M. K. Thornton and J. A. Potteiger, "Effects of Resistance Exercise Bouts of Different Intensities but Equal Work on EPOC," *Medicine and Science in Sports and Exercise* 34, no. 4 (April 2002): 715–22, PubMed PMID: 11932584.

12. K. Zahour and J. Porcari, "Dress Down, Shape Up," *ACE Fitness Matters* 10, no. 4 (2015).

13. C. I. Karageorghis, D. A. Mouzourides, D. L. Priest, T. A. Sasso, D. J. Morrish, and C. J. Walley, "Psychophysical and Ergogenic Effects of Synchronous Music During Treadmill Walking," *Journal of Sports Exercise Psychology* 31, no. 1 (February 2009): 18–36, PubMed PMID: 19325186.

14. "Hitting the gym? Scientists compile ultimate workout playlist," *Telegraph* (January 13, 2014) telegraph.co.uk.

15. N. A. Ratamess, J. G. Rosenberg, J. Kang, S. Sundberg, I. A. Izer, J. Levowsky, C. Rzeszutko, R. E. Ross, and A. D. Faigenbaum, "Acute Oxygen Uptake and Resistance Exercise Performance Using Different Rest Interval Lengths: The Influence Of Maximal Aerobic Capacity and Exercise Sequence," *Journal of Strength and Conditioning Research* 28, no. 7 (July 2014): 1875–88, doi: 10.1519/JSC.0000000000000485, PubMed PMID: 24714546.

16. K. K. Kattelmann, A. A. White, G. W. Greene, C. Byrd-Bredbenner, S. L. Hoerr, T. M. Horacek, T. Kidd, S. Colby, B. W. Phillips, M. M. Koenings, O. N. Brown, M. Olfert, K. P. Shelnutt, and J. S. Morrell, "Development of Young Adults Eating and Active for Health (YEAH) Internet-Based Intervention via a Community-Based Participatory Research Model," *Journal of Nutrition Education Behavior* 46, no. 2 (March–April 2014): S10–25, doi: 10.1016/j.jneb.2013.11.006.

17. A. W. Blanchfield, J. Hardy, H. M. De Morree, W. Staiano, and S. M. Marcora, "Talking Yourself out of Exhaustion: the Effects of Self-Talk on Endurance Performance," *Medicine and Science in Sports and Exercise* 46, no. 5 (2014): 998–1007, doi: 10.1249/MSS.0000000000000184. PubMed PMID: 24121242.

18. A. Poduri, D. L. Rateri, S. K. Saha, S, Saha, and A. Daugherty, "Citrullus lanatus 'Sentinel' (Watermelon) Extract Reduces Atherosclerosis in LDL Receptor-Deficient Mice," *Journal of Nutritional Biochemistry* 24, no. 5 (May 2013): 882–86, doi: 10.1016/j.jnutbio.2012.05.011.

19. M. P. Tarazona-Díaz, F. Alacid, M. Carrasco, I. Martínez, and E. Aguayo, "Watermelon Juice: Potential Functional Drink for Sore Muscle Relief in Athletes," *Journal of Agricultural and Food Chemistry* 61, no. 31 (August 2013): 7522–28, doi: 10.1021/jf400964r.

20. A. V. Nedeltcheva, J. M. Kilkus, J. Imperial, D. A. Schoeller, and P. D. Penev, "Insufficient Sleep Undermines Dietary Efforts to Reduce Adiposity," *Annals of Internal Medicine* 153, no. 7 (October 5, 2010): 435–41, doi: 10.7326/0003-4819-153-7-201010050-00006, PubMed PMID: 20921542

Bonus Chapter
24-Hour Damage Control—80 Ways to Kick Food Guilt to the Curb

1. K. J. Reid, G. Santostasi, K. G. Baron, J. Wilson, J. Kang, et al., "Timing and Intensity of Light Correlate with Body Weight in Adults," *PLOS ONE* 9, no. 4 (2014): e92251, doi: 10.1371/journal.pone.0092251,

2. *Amy Cuddy, Power Poser* (video), Game Changers, TIME Inc., March 19, 2012. time.com

3. A. Gallace, D. M. Torta, G. L. Moseley, and G. D. Iannetti, "The Analgesic Effect of Crossing the Arms," *Pain*. 152, no. 6 (June 2011): 1418–23, doi: 10.1016/j.pain.2011.02.029.

4. M. M. Bucchianeri and A. F. Corning, "An Experimental Test of Women's Body Dissatisfaction Reduction Through Self-Affirmation," *Applied Psychology: Health and Well-Being* 4 (2012): 188–201, doi: 10.1111/j.1758-0854.2012.01068.x.

5. IPCS, "Concise International Chemical Assessment Document No 5. Limonene," Geneva: WHO, 1998.

6. Cecilia Kang, "Google Crunches Data on Munching in Office," *Washington Post*, September 1, 2013. washingtonpost.com

7. M. Hatori, C. Vollmers, A. Zarrinpar, et al., "Time Restricted Feeding Without Reducing Caloric Intake Prevents Metabolic Diseases in Mice Fed a High Fat Diet," *Cell Metabolism* 15, no. 6 (2012): 848–60, doi: 10.1016/j.cmet.2012.04.019.

8. S. Brandhorst, I. Y. Choi, M. Wei, C. W. Cheng, S. Sedrakyan, G. Navarrete, L. Dubeau, L. P. Yap, R. Park, M. Vinciguerra, S. Di Biase, H. Mirzaei, M. G. Mirisola, P. Childress, L. Ji, S. Groshen, F. Penna, P. Odetti, L. Perin, P. S. Conti, Y. Ikeno, B. K. Kennedy, P. Cohen, T. E. Morgan, T. B. Dorff, and V. D. Longo, "A Periodic Diet That Mimics Fasting Promotes Multi-System Regeneration, Enhanced Cognitive Performance, and Healthspan," *Cell Metabolism* 22, no. 1 (July 2015): 86–99, doi: 10.1016/j.cmet.2015.05.012.

9. Ewa Jówko, "Green Tea Catechins and Sport Performance," *Antioxidants in Sport Nutrition* (Boca Raton, FL: CRC Press, 2014).

10. British Psychological Society, "Emotional Arousal Makes Us Better at Swearing," *ScienceDaily*, May 6, 2014.

11. Philip A. Kern, Brian S. Finlin, Beibei Zhu, Neda Rasouli, Robert E. McGehee, Philip M. Westgate, and Esther E. Dupont-Versteegden, "The Effects of Temperature and Seasons on Subcutaneous White Adipose Tissue in Humans: Evidence for Thermogenic Gene Induction," *The Journal of Clinical Endocrinology & Metabolism* 99, no. 12 (December 2014); jc.2014-2440, doi: 10.1210/jc.2014-2440.

12. W. G. Siems, F. J. van Kuijk, R. Maass, and R. Brenke, "Uric Acid and Glutathione Levels During Short-Term Whole Body Cold Exposure," *Free Radical Biology and Medicine* 16, no. 3 (March 1994): 299–305, PubMed PMID: 8063192.

13. "A Study Investigating the Relaxation Effects of the Music Track Weightless by Marconi Union," Mindlab International Ltd., PDF.

14. B. Hannover and U. Kühnen, "'The Clothing Makes the Self' Via Knowledge Activation," *Journal of Applied Social Psychology* 32 (2002): 2513–25, doi: 10.1111/j.1559-1816.2002.tb02754.x.

15. S. Craig Roberts, A. C. Little, A. Lyndon, J. Roberts, J. Havlicek, and R. L. Wright, "Manipulation of Body Odour Alters Men's Self-Confidence and Judgements of Their Visual Attractiveness by Women," *International Journal of Cosmetic Science* 31, no. 1 (February 2009): 47–54, doi: 10.1111/j.1468-2494.2008.00477.x, PubMed PMID: 19134127.

16. Javier T. Gonzalez, Rachel C. Veasey, Penny L. S. Rumbold, and Emma J. Stevenson, "Breakfast and Exercise Contingently Affect Postprandial Metabolism and Energy Balance in Physically Active Males," *British Journal of Nutrition* 110, no. 4 (2013): 721–32, doi: 10.1017/S0007114512005582.

17. T. L. Kraft and S. D. Pressman, "Grin and Bear It: The Influence of Manipulated Facial Expression on the Stress Response," *Psychological Science* 23, no. 11 (2012): 1372–78, doi: 10.1177/0956797612445312.

18. J. A. Greenberg and A. Geliebter, "Coffee, Hunger, and Peptide YY," *Journal of the American College of Nutrition* 31, no. 3 (June 2012): 160–66, PubMed PMID: 23204152.

19. L. Denti, I. Nilsson, I. Barbopoulos, L. Holmberg, M. Thulin, M. Wendeblad, et al., "Sweden's Largest Facebook Study: A Survey of 1000 Swedish Facebook Users," Gothenburg: Gothenburg Research Institute, 2012.

20. Penn State News, "Esteem Issues Determine How People Put Their Best Facebook Forward," 2013.

21. V. Stratton and A. Zalanowski, "Daily Music Listening Habits in College Students: Related Moods and Activities," *Psychology and Education Journal*, 2011.

22. M. Boschmann, J. Steiniger, U. Hille, J. Tank, F. Adams, A. M. Sharma, S. Klaus, F. C. Luft,and J. Jordan, "Water-Induced Thermogenesis," *Journal of Clinical Endocrinology and Metabolism* 88, no. 12 (December 2003): 6015–19, PubMed PMID: 14671205.

23. H. J. Oh and J. S. Park, [Effects of Hand Massage and Hand Holding on the Anxiety in Patients with Local Infiltration Anesthesia] [article in Korean], *Taehan Kanho Hakhoe Chi* 34, no. 6 (October 2004: 924–33, PubMed PMID: 15613828.

24. K. J. Sevits, E. L. Melanson, T. Swibas, et al., "Total Daily Energy Expenditure Is Increased Following a Single Bout of Sprint Interval Training," *Physiological Reports* 1, no. 5 (2013): e00131, doi: 10.1002/phy2.131.

25. H. Leidy, L. Ortineau, T. Rains, and K. Maki "Acute Effects of High Protein, Sausage and Egg-based Convenience Breakfast Meals on Postprandial Glucose Homeostasis in Healthy, Premenopausal Women," *FASEB* 28, no. 1, suppl. 381.6 (2014).

26. J. G. Wiese, M. G. Shlipak, and W. S. Browner, "The Alcohol Hangover," *Annals of Internal Medicine* 132 (2000): 897–902, doi: 10.7326/0003-4819-132-11-200006060-00008.

27. Jessica Gall Myrick, "Emotion Regulation, Procrastination, and Watching Cat Videos Online: Who Watches Internet Cats, Why, and to What Effect?," *Computers in Human Behavior* 52 (November 2015): 168-176, ISSN 0747-5632, http://dx.doi.org/10.1016/j.chb.2015.06.001.

28. A. Kong, S. A. Beresford, C. M. Alfano, K. E. Foster-Schubert, M. L. Neuhouser, D. B. Johnson, C. Duggan, C. Y. Wang, L. Xiao, C. E. Bain, and A. McTiernan, "Associations Between Snacking and Weight Loss and Nutrient Intake Among Postmenopausal Overweight to Obese Women in a Dietary Weight-Loss Intervention," *Journal of the American Dietetic Association* 111, no. 12 (December 2011): 1898-1903, doi: 10.1016/j.jada.2011.09.012, erratum in *Journal of the American Dietetic Association* 114, no. 6 (June 2014): 959, PubMed PMID: 22117666.

29. A. R. Hirsch and R. Gomez," "Weight Reduction Through Inhalation of Odorants," *Journal of Neurological and Orthopaedic Medicine and Surgery* 16 (1995): 26–31.

30. Iris W. Hung and Aparna A. Labroo, "From Firm Muscles to Firm Willpower: Understanding the Role of Embodied Cognition in Self-Regulation," *Journal of Consumer Research* (2011) available at SSRN: http://ssrn.com/abstract=1790324.

31. "10 Superfoods Healthier Than Kale," *Eat This, Not That!* eatthis.com.

32. J. A. Paniagua, A. Gallego de la Sacristana, I. Romero, A. Vidal-Puig, J. M. Latre, E. Sanchez, P. Perez-Martinez, J. Lopez-Miranda, and F. Perez-Jimenez, "Monounsaturated Fat-Rich Diet Prevents Central Body Fat Distribution and Decreases Postprandial Adiponectin Expression Induced by a Carbohydrate-Rich Diet in Insulin-Resistant Subjects," *Diabetes Care* 30, no. 7 (July 2007): 1717–23, published electronically March 23, 2007, PubMed PMID: 17384344.

33. "Leading Neuroscientist Says 'Viewing Art like Being in Love'" Art Fund, May 8, 2015. artfund.org

34. M. S. Buchowski, K. M. Majchrzak, K. Blomquist, K. Y. Chen, D. W. Byrne, and J. A. Bachorowski, "Energy Expenditure of Genuine Laughter," *International Journal of Obesity* (London) 31, no. 1 (January 2007):131-37, published electronically May 2, 2006, erratum in *International Journal of Obesity* (London) 38, no. 12 (December 2014): 1582, PubMed PMID: 16652129

35. C. A. Dow, S. B. Going, H. H. Chow, B. S. Patil, and C. A. Thomson, "The Effects of Daily Consumption of Grapefruit on Body Weight, Lipids, and Blood Pressure in Healthy, Overweight Adults," *Metabolism* 61, no. 7 (July 2012): 1026-35, doi: 10.1016/j. metabol.2011.12.004, published electronically February 2, 2012, PubMed PMID: 22304836.

36. I. D. Stephen, M. J. Law Smith, M. R. Stirrat, and D. I. Perrett, "Facial Skin Coloration Affects Perceived Health of Human Faces," *International Journal of Primatology* 30, no. 6 (2009): 845-57, doi: 10.1007/s10764-009-9380-z.

37. J. Nawijn, M. A. Marchand, R. Veenhoven, and A. J. Vingerhoets, "Vacationers Happier, but Most Not Happier After a Holiday," *Applied Research in Quality of Life* 5, no. 1 (March 2010): 35-47. Published electronically February 10, 2010, PubMed PMID: 20234864.

38. R. Dainese, J. Serra, F. Azpiroz, and J. R. Malagelada, "Influence of Body Posture on Intestinal Transit of Gas," *Gut* 52, no. 7 (July2003): 971-74, PubMed PMID: 12801953.

39. T. G. Allison, T. D. Miller, R. W. Squires, and G. T. Gau, "Cardiovascular Responses to Immersion in a Hot Tub in Comparison with Exercise in Male Subjects with Coronary Artery Disease," *Mayo Clinic Proceedings* 68, no. 1 (January 1993): 19-25, PubMed PMID: 8417250.

40. E. S. Mezzacappa, U. Arumugam, S. Y. Chen, T. R. Stein, M. Oz, and J. Buckle, "Coconut Fragrance and Cardiovascular Response to Laboratory Stress: Results of Pilot Testing," *Holistic Nursing Practice* 24, no. 6 (November-December 2010): 322-32, doi: 10.1097/ HNP.0b013e3181fbb89c.

41. Y. Maejima, Y. Iwasaki, Y. Yamahara, M. Kodaira, U. Sedbazar, and T. Yada, "Peripheral Oxytocin Treatment Ameliorates Obesity by Reducing Food Intake and Visceral Fat Mass," *Aging* (Albany, NY) 3, no. 12 (December 2011): 1169-77, PubMed PMID: 22184277.

42. David F. Hurlbert and Karen E. Whittaker, "The Role of Masturbation in Marital and Sexual Satisfaction: A Comparative Study of Female Masturbators and Nonmasturbators," *Journal of Sex Education & Therapy* 17, no. 4 (1991): 272-82.

43. Planned Parenthood Federation of America, *The Health Benefits of Sexual Expression*, white paper published in cooperation with the Society for Scientific Study of Sexuality, New York: Katherine Dexter McCormick Library, 2007.

44. M. Okla, I. Kang, D. M. Kim, V. Gourineni, N. Shay, L. Gu, and S. Chung, "Ellagic Acid Modulates Lipid Accumulation in Primary Human Adipocytes and Human Hepatoma Huh7 Cells via Discrete Mechanisms," *Journal of Nutritional Biochemistry* 26, no. 1 (January 2015): 82-90, doi: 10.1016/j.jnutbio.2014.09.010.

45. Trisha D. Scribbans, Jasmin K. Ma, Brittany A. Edgett, Kira A. Vorobej, Andrew S. Mitchell, Jason G.E. Zelt, Craig A. Simpson, Joe Quadrilatero, and Brendon J. Gurd, "Resveratrol Supplementation Does Not Augment Performance Adaptations or Fibre-Type–Specific Responses to High-Intensity Interval Training in Humans," *Applied Physiology, Nutrition, and Metabolism* 39, no. 11 (2014: 1305, doi: 10.1139/apnm-2014-0070

46. B. Wansink and K. van Ittersum, "Fast Food Restaurant Lighting and Music Can Reduce Calorie Intake and Increase Satisfaction," *Psychological Reports* 111, no. 1 (August 2012): 228–32, PubMed PMID: 23045865.

47. B. A. White, C. C. Horwath, and T. S. Conner, "Many Apples a Day Keep the Blues Away–Daily Experiences of Negative and Positive Affect and Food Consumption in Young Adults," *British Journal of Health Psychology* 18, no. 4 (November 2013): 782–98, doi: 10.1111/bjhp.12021.

48. X. Ying, X. Chen, S. Cheng, Y. Shen, and L. Peng, "Piperine Inhibits IL-Induced Expression of Inflammatory Mediators in Human Osteoarthritis Chondrocyte," *International Immunopharmacology* 17 (2013): 293–99.

49. Society for the Study of Ingestive Behavior, "Multiple Pieces of Food Are More Rewarding than an Equicaloric Single Piece of Food in Both Animals and Humans," *ScienceDaily*, July 10, 2012.

50. A. Franke, H. Harder, A. K. Orth, S. Zitzmann, and M. V. Singer, "Postprandial Walking but Not Consumption of Alcoholic Digestifs or Espresso Accelerates Gastric Emptying in Healthy Volunteers," *Journal of Gastrointestinal and Liver Diseases* 17, no. 1 (March 2008): 27–31, PMID: 18392240.

51. American Chemical Society, "Precise Reason for Health Benefits of Dark Chocolate: Thank Hungry Gut Microbes," *ScienceDaily*, March 18, 2014.

52. P. Lee, S, Smith, J. Linderman, A, B, Courville, R. J. Brychta, W. Dieckmann, C. D. Werner, K. Y. Chen, and F. S. Celi, "Temperature-Acclimated Brown Adipose Tissue Modulates Insulin Sensitivity in Humans," *Diabetes* 63, no. 11 (November 2014): 3686–98, doi: 10.2337/db14-0513, published electronically June 22, 2014, PubMed PMID: 24954193, PubMed Central PMCID: PMC4207391.

53. Tsutsui Yoshiro, "Weather and Individual Happiness," *Weather, Climate, and Society* 5 (2013): 70–82, doi: http://dx.doi.org/10.1175/WCAS-D-11-00052.1.

54. Debbie L. Cohen, Nancy Wintering, Victoria Tolles, Raymond R. Townsend, John T. Farrar, Mary Lou Galantino, and Andrew B. Newberg, "Cerebral Blood Flow Effects of Yoga Training: Preliminary Evaluation of 4 Cases," *Journal of Alternative and Complementary Medicine* 15, no. 1 (January 2009): 9–14, doi: 10.1089/acm.2008.0008.

55. K. Chandrasekhar, J. Kapoor, and S. Anishetty, "A Prospective, Randomized Double-Blind, Placebo-Controlled Study of Safety and Efficacy of a High-Concentration Full-Spectrum Extract of Ashwagandha Root in Reducing Stress and Anxiety in Adults," *Indian Journal of Psychological Medicine* 34, no. 3 (July 2012): 255–62, doi: 10.4103/0253-7176.106022, PubMed PMID: 23439798, PubMed Central PMCID: PMC3573577.

56. Biswajit Auddy et al., "A Standardized Withania somnifera Extract Significantly Reduces Stress-Related Parameters in Chronically Stressed Humans: A Double-Blind, Randomized, Placebo-Controlled Study," *Journal of the American Nutraceutical Association* 11, no. 1 (2008): 43–49.

57. Joshua J. Gooley, Kyle Chamberlain, Kurt A. Smith, Sat Bir S. Khalsa, Shantha M. W. Rajaratnam, Eliza Van Reen, Jamie M. Zeitzer, Charles A. Czeisler, and Steven W. Lockley, "Exposure to Room Light Before Bedtime Suppresses Melatonin Onset and Shortens Melatonin Duration in Humans," *Journal of Clinical Endocrinology and Metabolism* 96, no. 3 (March 2011): E463–E472. Published electronically December 30, 2010, doi: 10.1210/jc.2010-2098.

58. N. Goel, H. Kim, R. P. Lao, "An Olfactory Stimulus Modifies Nighttime Sleep in Young Men and Women," *Chronobiology International* 22, no. 5 (2005): 889–904, PMID: 16298774.

59. M. Schredl, D. Atanasova, K. Hörmann, J. T. Maurer, T. Hummel, and B. A. Stuck, "Information Processing During Sleep: The Effect of Olfactory Stimuli on Dream Content and Dream Emotions," *Journal of Sleep Research*, 18 (2009): 285–90, doi: 10.1111/j.1365-2869.2009.00737.x.

60. A. V. Nedeltcheva, J. M. Kilkus, J. Imperial, et al., "Insufficient Sleep Undermines Dietary Efforts to Reduce Adiposity," *Annals of Internal Medicine* 153 (2010): 435–41.

METRIC CONVERSIONS

The recipes in this book have not been tested with metric measurements, so some variations might occur.

Remember that the weight of dry ingredients varies according to the volume or density factor: 1 cup of flour weighs far less than 1 cup of sugar, and 1 tablespoon doesn't necessarily hold 3 teaspoons.

1. General Formulas for Metric Conversion

Ounces to grams:	ounces × 28.35 = grams
Grams to ounces:	grams × 0.035 = ounces
Pounds to grams:	pounds × 453.5 = grams
Pounds to kilograms:	pounds × 0.45 = kilograms
Cups to liters:	cups × 0.24 = liters
Fahrenheit to Celsius:	(°F − 32) × 5 ÷ 9 = °C
Celsius to Fahrenheit:	(°C × 9) ÷ 5 + 32 = °F

2. Linear Measurements

½ inch	=	1½ cm
1 inch	=	2½ cm
6 inches	=	15 cm
8 inches	=	20 cm
10 inches	=	25 cm
12 inches	=	30 cm
20 inches	=	50 cm

3. Volume (Dry) Measurements

¼ teaspoon	=	1 milliliter
½ teaspoon	=	2 milliliters
¾ teaspoon	=	4 milliliters
1 teaspoon	=	5 milliliters
1 tablespoon	=	15 milliliters
¼ cup	=	59 milliliters
⅓ cup	=	79 milliliters
½ cup	=	118 milliliters
⅔ cup	=	158 milliliters
¾ cup	=	77 milliliters
1 cup	=	225 milliliters
4 cups or 1 quart	=	1 liter
½ gallon	=	2 liters
1 gallon	=	4 liters

4. Volume (Liquid) Measurements

1 teaspoon	=	⅙ fluid ounce	=	5 milliliters
1 tablespoon	=	½ fluid ounce	=	15 milliliters
2 tablespoons	=	1 fluid ounce	=	30 milliliters
¼ cup	=	2 fluid ounces	=	60 milliliters
⅓ cup	=	2⅔ fluid ounces	=	79 milliliters
½ cup	=	4 fluid ounces	=	118 milliliters
1 cup or ½ pint	=	8 fluid ounces	=	250 milliliters
2 cups or 1 pint	=	16 fluid ounces	=	500 milliliters
4 cups or 1 quart	=	32 fluid ounces	=	1,000 milliliters
1 gallon	=	4 liters		

5. Oven Temperature Equivalents, Fahrenheit (F) and Celsius (C)

100°F	=	38°C
200°F	=	95°C
250°F	=	120°C
300°F	=	150°C
350°F	=	180°C
400°F	=	205°C
450°F	=	230°C

6. Weight (Mass) Measurements

1 ounce	=	30 grams		
2 ounces	=	55 grams		
3 ounces	=	85 grams		
4 ounces	=	¼ pound	=	125 grams
8 ounces	=	½ pound	=	240 grams
12 ounces	=	¾ pound	=	375 grams
16 ounces	=	1 pound	=	454 grams

Join Team Naughty Today!

Dear Naughty Girl,

Now that you've learned how to live your best, most sinfully delicious life–share it with someone! Join the thousands of women following the Naughty Diet on Facebook and Twitter for free content, community support, mouth-watering recipes and a shoulder to cry on, during those rare occasions when guilt returns, shame strikes, and you forget how awesome you are. (You are awesome!)

Team Naughty for life.

xo xo,
Melissa

ACKNOWLEDGMENTS

The Naughty Diet would not be possible without the support, advice, energy, and expertise of a large, talent pool: A special thank you to Dan Ambrosio, Jonathan Sainsbury, Kate Burke, Sean Maher and Miriam Riad at Perseus/Da Capo Lifelong Books.

To Joe Heroun, creative director of *Shape*, and his genius eye, for designing this book.

My infinite gratitude goes to Michael Freidson–*The Naughty Diet's* biological father, brilliant editor, and champion from day one. And to my special forces unit at Galvanized: George Karabotsos, Jon Hammond, Sean Bumgarner, Laura White, Linnea Zielinski, Dana Smith and Daniel McCarter, I salute you!

Also, a big thank you to the biggest agents in the industry: Jennifer Rudolph Walsh and Andy McNicol at WME. And to ubër editor Marnie Cochran at Random House, who loved the proposal and encouraged the book's publication.

To my long-suffering love, David Zinczenko–you make everything possible.

And finally, I thank my loving family. To my Mom and Dad, Burnett and Peter, for the gift of a happy childhood full of mischief. To my big brother Andrew, for his tough love–you only made me stronger! And thank you to my late sister, my guardian angel, my beloved Caroline, for blindly believing in me. Every day I am blessed by the love you lived.

INDEX

A

appetite suppressants, Naughty, 70

artificial sweeteners, 83

asparagus

Grilled Ratatouille Salad, 138

autonomic nervous system (ANS), 184

B

bacon or pancetta

Caramelized Bacon Popcorn, 143

Eggs in Purgatory, 128

Poached Egg over Frisée Salad, 132–133

bath, decadent, 191–192

beans

Brick Lane Curry, 145

beef

The Caffeinated Coffee-Rubbed Steak, 152

slow cooker chuck roast, 182

body, listening to, 58–60, 65–67

body-shaming. *See* shame

bourbon

Bourbon Caramel Sauce, 164

breakfast

Baked Egg with Mushrooms and Spinach, 126

Eggs in Purgatory, 128

French Toast Stuffed with Strawberries, 127

Green Goddess Smoothie, 123

World's Best Scrambled Eggs, 124–125

breathing, 184–186

C

calories, 3, 10, 83, 93–94, 185

carboload, 109

catechins, 173

cauliflower

Brick Lane Curry, 145

champagne

Champagne Gelée, 141

cheese

Caprese Tomato Towers, 130

Classic Chicken Parm, 148-149

Pizza with Arugula, Cherry Tomatoes, and Prosciutto, 154–155

chicken

Classic Chicken Parm, 148-149

The Roast Chicken, 146–147

chocolate

about, 65, 71, 175, 248

Chocolate-Covered Strawberries, 159

Chocolate Pudding with Olive Oil and Sea Salt, 158–159

Molten Chocolate Cake, 160–161

chocolate, white

Iced Berries Covered in Hot White Chocolate Sauce, 157

chronic comparers, 25

coconut milk

Brick Lane Curry, 145

coffee

about, 180

Affogato, 162

cortisol, 5–6, 238

cravings, 71

D

desserts

Affogato, 162

Berry Wine Sorbet, 168

Bourbon Caramel Sauce, 164

Chocolate-Covered

Strawberries, 159

Chocolate Pudding with Olive Oil and Sea Salt, 158–159

Fruitylicious Crumble, 166–167

Iced Berries Covered in Hot White Chocolate Sauce, 157

Molten Chocolate Cake, 160–161

Rosé Popsicles, 165

Strawberry Shortcake with Balsamic Vinegar, 163

Yogurt with honey and nuts, 170

diet sodas, 83

dinner

Brick Lane Curry, 145

The Caffeinated Coffee-Rubbed Steak, 152

Classic Chicken Parm, 148–149

Lemon-Stuffed Mediterranean Sea Bass Wrapped in Foil, 150

Pizza with Arugula, Cherry Tomatoes, and Prosciutto, 154–155

The Roast Chicken, 146–147

slow cooker chuck roast, 182

dopamine, 175

E

eggplant
Grilled Ratatouille Salad, 138
eggs
Baked Egg with Mushrooms and Spinach, 126
Eggs in Purgatory, 128
Poached Egg over Frisée Salad, 132–133
World's Best Scrambled Eggs, 124–125
ellagic acid, 193, 247
endorphins, 83, 208
enteric nervous system (ENS), 59–60
exercise, 215–220, 232–235

F

fasting, intermittent, 240
fat to sugar ratio, optimum, 83
fats, about, 169–170
"female Viagra" food, 172–175
fish
Lemon-Stuffed Mediterranean Sea Bass Wrapped in Foil, 150
Fitness Personality Quiz, 221–227
flavonoids, 175
food
aroma, importance of, 85
artificially sweetened, 83
changing language about, 43–44
changing thinking about, 204–207
enhancing pleasure of, 84–87
as "female Viagra," 172–175
food choice graph, 75
fresh, 91–92
loving, 120–121
nasty, 95–96
neurotic, 95–97
Pleasure Principles, 82
processed, 4–5, 83
quality, 77–79
SOUL, 81
top fifty Naughty foods, 99–112
truths, 83–84
variety, 62–65
food guilt
attitude toward, 13–17
causes of, 42–43
controlling, 57–59
defined, 41–42
forms of, 45–47
lessons from, 43
Naughty Diet and, xi
Naughty Quiz on, 49–55
post-indulgent-guilt, 87
releasing, 43–44, 47–48, 238–250
truths about, 40
weight loss and, 85
French fries, addictive nature of, 66
fruit
Avocado Dressing, 139
Avocado Toast with Red Pepper Flakes, 135
Berry Wine Sorbet, 168
Chocolate-Covered Strawberries, 159

Fruitylicious Crumble, 166–167
Green Goddess Smoothie, 123
Iced Berries Covered in Hot White Chocolate Sauce, 157
Rosé Popsicles, 165
Strawberry Shortcake with Balsamic Vinegar, 163

G

ghrelin, 66, 187

goddess greens, defined, 100

greens
Baked Egg with Mushrooms and Spinach, 126
Green Goddess juice, 170–171
kale chips, 142, 170
Poached Egg over Frisée Salad, 132–133

H

ham or Canadian bacon
Baked Egg with Mushrooms and Spinach, 126
healthy/sexy range, 29–30, 60
high-fructose corn syrup, 83
hunger, 68–69, 70
hydration, 239

I

indulging intelligently, 13
iron, 76, 174

K

kitchen equipment, 113–116

L

low blood sugar, 66
lunch
Avocado Dressing, 139
Avocado Toast with Red Pepper Flakes, 135
Caprese Tomato Towers, 130
Grilled Ratatouille Salad, 138
Poached Egg over Frisée Salad, 132–133
Quinoa Taboulé Salad, 136–137
Split Pea Soup, 134

M

mind games, 207

N

nasty, defined, 1–2
naughty, defined, 1–2
Naughty Cheats, 153, 159
Naughty Diet
5-point plan, 27–31
counting calories, 3, 10, 93–94
emotions and weight gain, 5–6
hunger, 4
mantras, 2, 6–7
processed food, 5
purpose of, xi–xiii

Naughty foods, 90–98

Naughty Nutrients, 169–171

Naughty Quiz on food guilt, 49–55

O

oenotherapy, defined, 194

P

P-Spot, 75–78

peas, split
  Split Pea Soup, 134

pizza
  Pizza with Arugula, Cherry Tomatoes, and Prosciutto, 154–155

Pleasure Principles, 82

polyphenols, 193

popcorn, 71, 143

Q

quality foods, 90–91

quinoa
  about, 170
  Quinoa Taboulé Salad, 136–137

R

relaxation, 178–179, 183–184, 200–201

resveratrol, 193, 194

rich, secret to becoming, 74

S

self-affirmations, 28

self-hypnosis, 208–212

serotonin, 71, 232

set point, 29–30

shame
  body shame, x–xi
  comparison with other women, 25–26
  creating positive body image, 27–31
  Naughty Diet and, 2, 5
  shame game, 18–19, 21–23
  slim shaming, xii, 32–37
  women and body-shaming, 24–26
  See also food guilt

sheets, buying, 187

skinny fat, 11–12

sleep, 67, 186–190

snacks
  Caramelized Bacon Popcorn, 143
  kale chips, 142, 170
  suggestions, 142

SOUL food, 81

squash
  Brick Lane Curry, 145
  Grilled Ratatouille Salad, 138

squirrel food, defined, 105

stress, 183–184

subconscious, retraining, 210–215

superseeds, 111

T

tea, ashwagandha, 249

tea, green, 173, 228, 240

tomatoes
  Brick Lane Curry, 145
  Caprese Tomato Towers, 130
  Pizza with Arugula, Cherry Tomatoes, and Prosciutto, 154–155

tryptophan, 188

W

weight, losing, 83–85, 180–182, 188–190

weight fluctuations, 39–40, 60

wine
  benefits of, 173, 192–194
  Berry Wine Sorbet, 168
  descriptive terms, 199–201
  enjoyment of, 86
  Rosé Popsicles, 165
  types of, 195–199

workout, 232-235

workout, increasing effectiveness of, 228–231

Y

yogurt
  Yogurt with honey and nuts, 170